Understanding the Personality Inventory for DSM-5 (PID-5)

Understanding the Personality Inventory for DSM-5 (PID-5)

Kristian E. Markon, Ph.D.

Andrea Fossati, Ph.D.

Antonella Somma, Ph.D.

Robert F. Krueger, Ph.D.

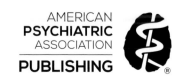

AMERICAN
PSYCHIATRIC
ASSOCIATION
PUBLISHING

Copyright © 2024 American Psychiatric Association Publishing
ALL RIGHTS RESERVED
First Edition
Manufactured in the United States of America on acid-free paper
28 27 26 25 24   5 4 3 2 1

American Psychiatric Association Publishing
800 Maine Avenue SW, Suite 900
Washington, DC 20024-2812
www.appi.org

Library of Congress Cataloging-in-Publication Data
Names: Markon, Kristian, author. | Fossati, Andrea, 1963- author. | Somma, Antonella, author. | Krueger, Robert F., author. | American Psychiatric Association Publishing, issuing body.
Title: Understanding the personality inventory for DSM-5 (PID-5) / Kristian E. Markon, Andrea Fossati, Antonella Somma, Robert F. Krueger.
Description: First edition. | Washington, D.C. : American Psychiatric Association Publishing, [2024] | Includes bibliographical references and index.
Identifiers: LCCN 2023032665 (print) | LCCN 2023032666 (ebook) | ISBN 9781615375110 (paperback ; alk. paper) | ISBN 9781615375127 (ebook)
Subjects: MESH: Diagnostic and statistical manual of mental disorders. 5th ed | Personality Inventory | Personality Assessment | Personality Disorders--diagnosis
Classification: LCC RC473.P56 (print) | LCC RC473.P56 (ebook) | NLM WM 145.5.M6 | DDC 616.85/81075--dc23/eng/20231108
LC record available at https://lccn.loc.gov/2023032665
LC ebook record available at https://lccn.loc.gov/2023032666

British Library Cataloguing in Publication Data
A CIP record is available from the British Library.

Contents

ABOUT THE AUTHORS

Kristian E. Markon, Ph.D., is Research Scientist in the Department of Psychology at the University of Minnesota in Minneapolis, Minnesota.

Andrea Fossati, Ph.D., is Professor of Clinical Psychology in the School of Psychology at Vita-Salute San Raffaele University in Milan, Italy.

Antonella Somma, Ph.D., is Assistant Professor of Clinical Psychology in the School of Psychology at Vita-Salute San Raffaele University in Milan, Italy.

Robert F. Krueger, Ph.D., is Distinguished McKnight University Professor and Hathaway Distinguished Professor in the Department of Psychology at the University of Minnesota in Minneapolis, Minnesota; Co-Editor of the *Journal of Personality Disorders*; and former Chairperson of the U.S. NIH/CSR Social, Personality and Interpersonal Processes study section.

DISCLOSURE OF INTERESTS

Kristian E. Markon, Ph.D., is a coauthor of the PID-5. PID-5 is the intellectual property of the American Psychiatric Association, and Dr. Markon does not receive royalties or any other compensation from publication or administration of the inventory.

Andrea Fossati, Ph.D., translated the PID-5 into Italian language and is a coauthor of the Italian PID-5 Manual. Dr. Fossati provides consulting services to aid users of the PID-5 in the interpretation of test scores and does not receive royalties or any other compensation from publication or administration of the PID-5.

Antonella Somma, Ph.D., is a coauthor of the Italian PID-5 Manual. Dr. Somma provides consulting services to aid users of the PID-5 in the interpretation of test scores and does not receive royalties or any other compensation from publication or administration of the PID-5.

Robert F. Krueger, Ph.D., is a coauthor of the PID-5 and provides consulting services to aid users of the PID-5 in the interpretation of test scores. PID-5 is the intellectual property of the American Psychiatric Association, and Dr. Krueger does not receive royalties or any other compensation from publication or administration of the inventory.

PREFACE

With this book, we provide background and information about the Personality Inventory for DSM-5 (PID-5) and its properties for use in research and applied practice. Since the official release of the PID-5 in 2012, interest in this assessment measure has grown dramatically both in the United States and around the world, spawning an impressive amount of research. The PID-5 was developed as a free, easily administered measure of the domains and traits of personality pathology as described in Criterion B of the Alternative Model for Personality Disorders (AMPD) in the *Diagnostic and Statistical Manual of Mental Disorders,* 5th Edition (DSM-5; American Psychiatric Association 2013). In our opinion, the success of the PID-5 in generating sound, realistic descriptions of personality pathology has provided a good foundation for adoption of the AMPD and other modern approaches to clinical assessment and treatment planning. In this book, we hope to convey what has contributed to increasing use of the PID-5 in the United States and across the world. Assessment relying on the PID-5 implies a shift from personality diagnosis per se—trying to fit an individual's personal experience into diagnostic categories—to ascertaining a profile reflecting an individual's unique experiences and behaviors. Using the PID-5 and AMPD more broadly implies the adoption in routine clinical assessment of a more individualized, person-centered approach to understanding the patient's specific concerns and characteristics. This approach may also help clinicians adopt a holistic understanding of the problems of a patient, with reference to current presentation as well as the patient's history and progression. The instrument might help both clinicians and their individual patients make sense of acute symptoms and transient problems (see also DeYoung et al. 2022) and predict the possibility of problematic reactions to stressors and other circumstances (e.g., separations, work problems, house moving, treatment discontinuation).

This approach to assessment also may promote the identification of individual developmental pathways that in their atypical form lead to dysfunctional personality patterns that might be studied longitudinally. Available evidence on the continuities (e.g., Suzuki et al. 2015,

2019; Wright et al. 2017) between nonclinically derived (i.e., Five Factor Model dimensions and facets) and pathological personality traits (e.g., PID-5 domains and traits) may prove useful when translating available evidence on the development of personality traits into research on atypical developmental trajectories that lead to personality pathology. Along these lines, the PID-5 in some form may be a viable instrument for early identification of emerging personality dysfunction in adolescence without the stigmatizing or labeling bias of traditional approaches to personality disorder assessment, as initial research seems to indicate (e.g., De Fruyt and De Clercq 2014; Fossati and Somma 2021; Sharp et al. 2021). Further research is needed to develop and characterize the PID-5 for use in younger populations and to obtain a better understanding of how personality pathology is best assessed in that developmental period, including the role of family and other individuals in adolescents' lives.

Understanding the influences on an individual patient's responses is critical to accurate interpretation of their scores in clinical settings. Ambivalence about testing, inattention, motivations to present oneself positively or negatively, and pressures to otherwise convey certain impressions in testing are all examples of extraneous influences on test scores other than the traits of interest. Emerging evidence and resources, reviewed throughout this book, provide mechanisms for assessing sources of invalidity in testing and for integrating different sources of information in the assessment process to compile a more complete, comprehensive interpretation of patients' scores and responses. Nevertheless, more research is needed to better characterize threats to validity of individual responses and how to assess these threats. Additional information on how underreporting indexes generalize across populations and settings is needed, for example, as is a better understanding of how different forms of impression management affect responding. The informant report form provides another mechanism for addressing sources of invalidity, but informants themselves have their own reasons for responding randomly or in a biased manner; more research is needed to develop validity indexes for informant report and to better understand how to integrate different sources of information about individuals' personality-related problems.

These concerns notwithstanding, a substantial body of data has now provided evidence for the reliability and validity of the PID-5. Meta-analyses (e.g., Somma et al. 2019) have convincingly shown that the factor structure of the PID-5 trait scales replicates across several different countries, languages, and cultures. This finding is helpful in integrating results from studies carried out in different countries and cultural contexts, as well as in facilitating clinical communication and development, but also supports the generalizability of PID-5 interpretation across different populations more broadly. At the same time, there is much to be done—these initial findings across different contexts represent a starting point for further investigating the generalizability and application of the PID-5. For example, future research and clinical efforts should continue to delineate the properties of the PID-5 in different sociodemographic populations, examine the generalizability and properties of empirically based score thresholds in different populations, evaluate the validity and use of the PID-5 in assessing special populations (e.g., refugees, migrants), and review the development of normative information for people from minority or disadvantaged backgrounds. All these issues are important as future targets for both clinicians and researchers interested in the PID-5.

As a final prefatory remark, we would like to underscore that the publication of the PID-5 has stimulated incredible research and clinical efforts promoting collaboration between clinicians and researchers who come from different part of the world, work in different fields, and have different backgrounds. We hope that this book will encourage curious readers to further explore dimensional assessment of personality psychopathology (Clark et al. 2015).

REFERENCES

American Psychiatric Association: Diagnostic and Statistical Manual of Mental Disorders, 5th Edition. Washington, DC, American Psychiatric Association, 2013

Clark LA, Vanderbleek EN, Shapiro JL, et al: The brave new world of personality disorder-trait specified: effects of additional definitions on coverage, prevalence, and comorbidity. Psychopathol Rev 2(1):52–82, 2015 26097740

De Fruyt F, De Clercq B: Antecedents of personality disorder in childhood and adolescence: toward an integrative developmental model. Annu Rev Clin Psychol 10:449–476, 2014 24471374

DeYoung CG, Chmielewski M, Clark LA, et al: The distinction between symptoms and traits in the Hierarchical Taxonomy of Psychopathology (HiTOP). J Pers 90(1):20–33, 2022 32978977

Fossati A, Somma A: The assessment of personality pathology in adolescence from the perspective of the Alternative DSM-5 Model for Personality Disorder. Curr Opin Psychol 37:39–43, 2021 32827876

Sharp C, Chanen A, Cavelti M: Personality challenges in young people: from description to action. Curr Opin Psychol 37:v–ix, 2021 33741118

Somma A, Krueger RF, Markon KE, et al: The replicability of the Personality Inventory for DSM-5 domain scale factor structure in U.S. and non-U.S. samples: a quantitative review of the published literature. Psychol Assess 31(7):861–877, 2019 30883152

Suzuki T, Samuel DB, Pahlen S, et al: DSM-5 Alternative Personality Disorder Model traits as maladaptive extreme variants of the Five-Factor Model: an item-response theory analysis. J Abnorm Psychol 124(2):343–354, 2015 25665165

Suzuki T, South SC, Samuel DB, et al: Measurement invariance of the DSM-5 Section III pathological personality trait model across sex. Personal Disord 10(2):114–122, 2019 29952589

Wright ZE, Pahlen S, Krueger RF: Genetic and environmental influences on Diagnostic and Statistical Manual of Mental Disorders-Fifth Edition (DSM-5) maladaptive personality traits and their connections with normative personality traits. J Abnorm Psychol 126(4):416–428, 2017 28368150

ACKNOWLEDGMENTS

We are deeply grateful to the editorial team at American Psychiatric Association Publishing for supporting our project and providing us with constructive suggestions and editorial input. We are also grateful to the American Psychiatric Association for funding the collection of normative data, without which this book would not be possible. We would like to take the opportunity to thank Giulia Gialdi, Linda Boscaro, Arianna De Ciechi, Chiara Arioli, Valeria Mariani, and Alessia Di Tommaso for their contributions in collecting relevant material at the initial stages of this book and also would like to acknowledge Raffaello Cortina Editore for increasing interest in and disseminating information about the Personality Inventory for DSM-5 (PID-5) in Italy. Finally, we wish to thank all the clinicians who rely on the PID-5 in working with their patients.

CHAPTER 1

Development and Origins of the PID-5

PERSONALITY INVENTORY FOR DSM-5

The Personality Inventory for DSM-5 (PID-5; American Psychiatric Association 2013; Krueger et al. 2012) is a measure developed for the assessment of the Alternative Model for Personality Disorders Personality Trait Model (AMPD-TM) listed in Section III of the fifth edition of the *Diagnostic and Statistical Manual of Mental Disorders* (DSM-5; American Psychiatric Association 2013). Specifically, the PID-5 operationalizes the personality trait aspect of the DSM-5 Section III personality disorder model (i.e., Criterion B). Accordingly, it allows for assessment of 25 dysfunctional personality traits, which represent specific elements of maladaptive personality variation, and 5 broad dysfunctional personality domains that capture the higher-order structural organization of the 25 specific traits. The AMPD definitions of PID-5 domains and traits are listed in Table 1–1.

Although the PID-5 is usually referred to as a single measure, it may be more accurate to consider the PID-5 as a family of instruments developed starting with the 220-item self-report version of the PID-5. Consistent with historical patterns in personality assessment, the PID-5 was initially constructed as a self-report instrument and was later expanded to other forms. The need for a multimethod perspective in personality assessment and the need to meet assessment requirements in contexts

Table 1–1. Description of the Personality Inventory for DSM-5 domains and traits

Domain	Definition
Negative affect	Frequent and intense experiences of high levels of a wide range of negative emotions (e.g., anxiety, depression, guilt/shame, worry, anger) and their behavioral (e.g., self-harm) and interpersonal (e.g., dependency) manifestations
Emotional lability	Instability of emotional experiences and mood; emotions that are easily aroused, intense, and/or out of proportion to events and circumstances
Anxiousness	Feelings of nervousness, tenseness, or panic in reaction to diverse situations; frequent worry about the negative effects of past unpleasant experiences and future negative possibilities; feeling fearful and apprehensive about uncertainty; expecting the worst to happen
Restricted affectivity	Little reaction to emotionally arousing situations; constricted emotional experience and expression; indifference and aloofness in normatively engaging situations
Separation insecurity	Fears of being alone due to rejection by and/or separation from significant others, based in a lack of confidence in one's ability to care for oneself, both physically and emotionally
Hostility	Persistent or frequent angry feelings; anger or irritability in response to minor slights and insults; mean, nasty, or vengeful behavior
Perseveration	Persistence at tasks or in a particular way of doing things long after the behavior has ceased to be functional or effective; continuance of the same behavior despite repeated failures or clear reasons for stopping
Submissiveness	Adaptation of one's behavior to the actual or perceived interests and desires of others even when doing so is antithetical to one's own interests, needs, or desires
Detachment	Avoidance of socioemotional experience, including both withdrawal from interpersonal interactions (ranging from casual daily interactions to friendships to intimate relationships) and restricted affective experience and expression, particularly limited hedonic capacity

Table 1–1. Description of the Personality Inventory for DSM-5 domains and traits *(continued)*

Domain	Definition
Withdrawal	Preference for being alone to being with others; reticence in social situations; avoidance of social contacts and activity; lack of initiation of social contact
Anhedonia	Lack of enjoyment from, engagement in, or energy for life's experiences; deficits in the capacity to feel pleasure or take interest in things
Depressivity	Feelings of being down, miserable, and/or hopeless; difficulty recovering from such moods; pessimism about the future; pervasive shame and/or guilt; feelings of inferior self-worth; thoughts of suicide and suicidal behavior
Intimacy avoidance	Avoidance of close or romantic relationships, interpersonal attachments, and intimate sexual relationships
Suspiciousness	Expectations of and sensitivity to signs of interpersonal ill intent or harm; doubts about loyalty and fidelity of others; feelings of being mistreated, used, and/or persecuted by others
Antagonism	Behaviors that put the individual at odds with other people, including an exaggerated sense of self-importance and a concomitant expectation of special treatment, as well as a callous antipathy toward others, encompassing both an unawareness of others' needs and feelings and a readiness to use others in the service of self-enhancement
Manipulativeness	Use of subterfuge to influence or control others; use of seduction, charm, glibness, or ingratiation to achieve one's ends
Deceitfulness	Dishonesty and fraudulence; misrepresentation of self; embellishment or fabrication when relating events
Grandiosity	Believing that one is superior to others and deserves special treatment; self-centeredness; feelings of entitlement; condescension toward others
Attention seeking	Engaging in behavior designed to attract notice and to make oneself the focus of others' attention and admiration

Table 1–1. Description of the Personality Inventory for DSM-5 domains and traits *(continued)*

Domain	Definition
Callousness	Lack of concern for feelings or problems of others; lack of guilt or remorse about the negative or harmful effects of one's actions on others
Disinhibition	Orientation toward immediate gratification, leading to impulsive behavior driven by current thoughts, feelings, and external stimuli, without regard for past learning or consideration of future consequences
Irresponsibility	Disregard for and failure to honor financial and other obligations or commitments; lack of respect for and lack of follow-through on agreements and promises; carelessness with others' property
Impulsivity	Acting on the spur of the moment in response to immediate stimuli; acting on a momentary basis without plan or consideration of outcomes; difficulty establishing and following plans; a sense of urgency and self-harming behavior under emotional distress
Risk taking	Engagement in dangerous, risky, and potentially self-damaging activities, unnecessarily and without regard to consequences; lack of concern for one's limitations and denial of the reality of personal danger; reckless pursuit of goals regardless of the level of risk involved
Rigid perfectionism	Rigid insistence on everything being flawless, perfect, and without errors or faults, including one's own and others' performance; sacrificing of timeliness to ensure correctness in every detail; believing that there is only one right way to do things; difficulty changing ideas and/or viewpoint; preoccupation with details, organization, and order
Distractibility	Difficulty concentrating and focusing on tasks; attention easily diverted by extraneous stimuli; difficulty maintaining goal-focused behavior, including both planning and completing tasks
Psychoticism	Exhibiting a wide range of culturally incongruent odd, eccentric, or unusual behaviors and cognitions, including both process (e.g., perception, dissociation) and content (e.g., beliefs)

Table 1–1. Description of the Personality Inventory for DSM-5 domains and traits *(continued)*

Domain	Definition
Unusual beliefs and experiences	Belief that one has unusual abilities, such as mind reading, telekinesis, thought-action fusion, or unusual experiences of reality, including hallucination-like experiences
Eccentricity	Odd, unusual, or bizarre behavior, appearance, and/or speech; having strange and unpredictable thoughts; saying unusual or inappropriate things
Cognitive and perceptual dysregulation	Odd or unusual thought processes and experiences, including depersonalization, derealization, and dissociative experiences; mixed sleep-wake state experiences; thought-control experiences.

Source. Adapted from American Psychiatric Association: *Diagnostic and Statistical Manual of Mental Disorders*, 5th Edition. Arlington, VA, American Psychiatric Association, 2013, pp. 779–781. Used with permission. Copyright © 2013 American Psychiatric Association.

where self-report may be a suboptimal choice (e.g., forensic settings) led to the development of clinician- and informant-rated versions of the PID-5 (different forms of the PID-5 are the focus of Chapter 3, "The PID-5s").

DEVELOPMENT OF THE PID-5

The primary objective for constructing the PID-5 was to provide an empirical basis for the organization of personality disorder features in the DSM-5 classification of personality disorder variables. The history of the PID-5 is rooted in the work done by the Personality and Personality Disorders Work Group and was meant to implement an empirically based, dimensional approach to personality disorder classification. The PID-5 was developed according to a hypothetico-deductive process (Cattell 1978; see Krueger 2019). Although the revision process leading to the DSM-5 AMPD is not the focus of the current manual and is documented elsewhere (e.g., Zachar et al. 2016), it may be relevant in that the logic behind the development of the AMPD-TM was based on the idea that clinical expertise represents a suitable starting point for identifying constructs relevant to understanding personality pathology. Operationalization of these concepts should follow to allow for data collection, an essential step in providing empirical support to the resulting model of personality. This process was the foundation for the development of the PID-5 (see Krueger 2019), which now represents the most direct and widely used approach to assess the AMPD-TM.

Identification of a Personality Trait Model Suitable for DSM-5

The construction of the AMPD-TM started with a review of models and measures of maladaptive personality traits, with a focus on furthering work by Widiger and Simonsen (2005) in which four broad domains were identified as common across different models of personality. Importantly, Widiger and Simonsen (2005) suggested that clinicians should focus their attention on the maladaptive variants of the personality traits because they are of most relevance to capturing the cornerstones of personality pathology. Specifically, the first dimension is characterized by withdrawal, isolation, and introversion, corresponding to the lower extreme of the Five Factor Model (FFM) extraversion personality trait. The second broad personality dimension contrasts deceptive, manipulative, or antagonistic interpersonal relatedness with agreeableness, modesty, and empathy; this personality dimension markedly overlaps with the FFM agreeableness versus antagonism construct (Widiger and Simonsen 2005). Additionally, Widiger and Simonsen (2005) identified a third domain of conscientiousness versus disinhibition, which contrasts being disciplined, conscientious, and achievement oriented with being irresponsible, impulsive, and negligent (i.e., conscientiousness vs. disinhibition in FFM terms). The fourth dimension contrasts the intensity and frequency of anxiety, depression, and anger with the experience of emotional stability and calm (i.e., FFM neuroticism vs. emotional stability). Finally, following Harkness et al.'s (1995) five-factor model of dysfunctional personality, the inclusion of a fifth domain, psychoticism, was proposed, reflecting difficulties with cognitive disorganization and unusual behavior and perceptual experiences.

Item Pool Development and Measure Construction

As described extensively by Krueger et al. (2012), in the earliest phase of the PID-5 development process, the Personality and Personality Disorders Work Group members were encouraged to make a list of the dysfunctional personality features they found to be most clinically relevant in their work with patients with personality disorders. This process resulted in a list of 37 specific facets. Following this initial stage, definitions of each of the traits were provided by the authors of the PID-5 first validation study (Krueger et al. 2012), and an initial item pool based on these descriptions was constructed. This allowed an empirical investigation of this initial item pool.

The initial measure construction took place over the course of two rounds of data collection. Round 1 involved a sample of 762 community-dwelling participants who had sought treatment for mental health issues, drawn from a representative survey panel of the U.S. population. In order to evaluate the ability of the initial item pool to measure the 37 initial facets, round 1 participants were administered 296 items, with four Likert response options from "very false or often false" to "very true or often true." On the basis of the results of the first round of data collection, the initial item pool was refined empirically, relying on both classical test theory and item response theory methods. Round 2 involved a total of 366 participants, sampled with the same selection and weighting scheme used in round 1, who completed a total of 316 items: 231 items from round 1 and 85 new ones. The results of the second round of data collection suggested reduction of the initial 37 traits to 25, combining facets that were highly redundant (e.g., depressivity, guilt and shame, low self-esteem, pessimism, and self-harm were collapsed in the depressivity trait facet; see the definition of depressivity in Table 1–1) as suggested by item-level within-domain exploratory factor analysis.

The 220-Item Version of the PID-5

The measure resulting from both rounds of data collection, the PID-5, is composed of 220 items, and its basic psychometric properties were assessed in a third round of data collection from a representative sample of the U.S. population (N=264) that was specifically designed to examine the 25 identified facets or specific traits. Factor analysis results showed that these 25 specific traits could be empirically organized around 5 broad dimensions or domains of personality. These broad domains were termed *negative affect, detachment, antagonism, disinhibition,* and *psychoticism* (see Table 1–1). PID-5 Emotional Lability, Anxiousness, Restricted Affectivity, Separation Insecurity, Hostility, Perseveration, and Submissiveness scores constitute indicators in the negative affect domain; PID-5 Withdrawal, Anhedonia, Depressivity, Intimacy Avoidance, and Suspiciousness scores are in the detachment domain; Manipulativeness, Deceitfulness, Grandiosity, Attention Seeking, and Callousness scores are in the antagonism domain; Irresponsibility, Impulsivity, Rigid Perfectionism, Distractibility, and Risk Taking scores are in the disinhibition domain; and Unusual Beliefs and Experiences, Eccentricity, and Cognitive and Perceptual Dysregulation scores are in the psychoticism domain.

REMARKS ON THE PID-5 AND ITS DEVELOPMENT

The approach used to develop the PID-5 was grounded in existing models of personality (e.g., Clark 2007; Costa and Widiger 2002; Harkness et al. 1995; Watson et al. 2008), but it is important to note that the generation of the PID-5 (and, consequently, of the AMPD-TM model) was an empirical enterprise. As a result, as might be predicted, the higher-order domains constituting the AMPD-TM parallel other empirically based personality and personality disorder trait models in the literature. For instance, Suzuki and colleagues (2015), relying on item response theory, showed that the PID-5 and a widely used FFM measure (the International Personality Item Pool–NEO; IPIP-NEO) are both measures of neuroticism, extraversion, agreeableness, and conscientiousness. Similarly, isomorphism between the PID-5 domains and the Personality Psychopathology Five (PSY-5) domains (e.g., Anderson et al. 2013), the Dimensional Assessment of Personality Pathology—Basic Questionnaire (DAPP-BQ; e.g., Gutiérrez et al. 2020), and the Schedule for Nonadaptive and Adaptive Personality (SNAP) domains (e.g., Crego and Widiger 2020) also has been demonstrated. In addition, Hopwood and colleagues (2013) showed connections between the AMPD-TM, as assessed by the PID-5, and a range of clinical variables as instantiated in the Personality Assessment Inventory (PAI; Morey 1991).

It should be observed that the PID-5 was meant to assess traits that largely account for individual differences in the expression of personality disorder (e.g., Morey and Skodol 2013; Samuel et al. 2013; Watters et al. 2019). Since its release, which preceded the publication of DSM-5, the PID-5 has been highly generative, promoting a rapid increase in the literature assessing different aspects of the AMPD-TM (see Chapter 2, "Basic Measurement Properties and Validity of the PID-5 Across Populations").

REFERENCES

American Psychiatric Association: Diagnostic and Statistical Manual of Mental Disorders, 5th Edition. Washington, DC, American Psychiatric Association, 2013
Anderson JL, Sellbom M, Bagby RM, et al: On the convergence between PSY-5 domains and PID-5 domains and facets: implications for assessment of DSM-5 personality traits. Assessment 20(3):286–294, 2013 23297369

Cattell RB: The Scientific Use of Factor Analysis in Behavioral and Life Sciences. New York, Plenum, 1978

Clark LA: Assessment and diagnosis of personality disorder: perennial issues and an emerging reconceptualization. Annu Rev Psychol 58:227–257, 2007 16903806

Costa PT Jr, Widiger TA: Personality Disorders and the Five-Factor Model of Personality, 2nd Edition. Washington, DC, American Psychological Association, 2002

Crego C, Widiger TA: The convergent, discriminant, and structural relationship of the DAPP-BQ and SNAP with the ICD-11, DSM-5, and FFM trait models. Psychol Assess 32(1):18–28, 2020 31328932

Gutiérrez F, Ruiz J, Peri JM, et al: Toward an integrated model of pathological personality traits: common hierarchical structure of the PID-5 and the DAPP-BQ. J Pers Disord 34(Suppl C):25–39, 2020 31210573

Harkness AR, McNulty JL, Ben-Porath YS: The Personality Psychopathology Five (PSY-5): constructs and MMPI-2 scales. Psychol Assess 7:104–114, 1995

Hopwood CJ, Wright AGC, Krueger RF, et al: DSM-5 pathological personality traits and the personality assessment inventory. Assessment 20(3):269–285, 2013 23610235

Krueger RF: Criterion B of the AMPD and the interpersonal, multivariate, and empirical paradigms of personality assessment, in The DSM-5 Alternative Model for Personality Disorders: Integrating Multiple Paradigms of Personality Assessment. Edited by Hopwood CJ, Mulay AL, Waugh MH. New York, Taylor & Francis, 2019, pp 60–76

Krueger RF, Derringer J, Markon KE, et al: Initial construction of a maladaptive personality trait model and inventory for DSM-5. Psychol Med 42(9):1879–1890, 2012 22153017

Morey LC: Professional Manual for the Personality Assessment Inventory. Odessa, FL, Psychological Assessment Resources, 1991

Morey LC, Skodol AE: Convergence between DSM-IV-TR and DSM-5 diagnostic models for personality disorder: evaluation of strategies for establishing diagnostic thresholds. J Psychiatr Pract 19(3):179–193, 2013 23653075

Samuel DB, Hopwood CJ, Krueger RF, et al: Comparing methods for scoring personality disorder types using maladaptive traits in DSM-5. Assessment 20(3):353–361, 2013 23588686

Suzuki T, Samuel DB, Pahlen S, et al: DSM-5 alternative personality disorder model traits as maladaptive extreme variants of the five-factor model: an item-response theory analysis. J Abnorm Psychol 124(2):343–354, 2015 25665165

Watson D, Clark LA, Chmielewski M: Structures of personality and their relevance to psychopathology, II: further articulation of a comprehensive unified trait structure. J Pers 76(6):1545–1586, 2008 19012658

Watters CA, Bagby RM, Sellbom M: Meta-analysis to derive an empirically based set of personality facet criteria for the Alternative DSM-5 Model for Personality Disorders. Pers Disord 10(2):97–104, 2019 30520649

Widiger TA, Simonsen E: Alternative dimensional models of personality disorder: finding a common ground. J Pers Disord 19(2):110–130, 2005 15899712

Zachar P, Krueger RF, Kendler KS: Personality disorder in DSM-5: an oral history. Psychol Med 46(1):1–10, 2016 26482368

CHAPTER 2

Basic Measurement Properties and Validity of the PID-5 Across Populations

Since its release, the DSM-5 Alternative Model for Personality Disorders (AMPD; American Psychiatric Association 2013) has prompted a rapidly growing amount of research. Much of this research has focused on AMPD Criterion B (i.e., pathological personality traits) and the measure that was explicitly designed to assess it, the Personality Inventory for DSM-5 (PID-5). Although there are many possible reasons for this growth in interest, it could be argued that the availability of an easy-to-administer, free, and readily translated self-report measure has contributed to the proliferation of research studies on the AMPD as well as on the PID-5 in the United States and across the world.

BASIC MEASUREMENT PROPERTIES IN ADULTS AND ADOLESCENTS

The AMPD's innovative approach to pathological personality conceptualization aimed to foster connections between research and clinical practice and to help clinicians understand dysfunctional personality from the perspective of atypical development of normative personality dimensions. It is noteworthy that just 1 year after the publication of the PID-5 (Krueger et al. 2012), dysfunctional personality domains and traits assessed through the PID-5 were shown to be highly correlated with clinician-rated counterparts in a sample of 109 individuals receiving outpatient mental health treatment (Few et al. 2013). The PID-5 traits and domains also proved useful in accounting for DSM-IV (American Psychiatric Association 1994) personality disorder diagnoses and internalizing symptoms (i.e., anxiety and depression) and externalizing behaviors (i.e., alcohol and drug use).

In U.S. studies, the PID-5 demonstrates generally adequate psychometric properties across samples and populations, such as in college student, community, psychiatric, and forensic samples (e.g., Dunne et al. 2018; Few et al. 2013; Gore and Widiger 2013; Hopwood et al. 2012; Quilty et al. 2013; Wright et al. 2015). Specifically, the PID-5 domain and scale scores show strong internal consistency, a replicable five-factor structure, convergence with existing personality instruments, and expected associations with meaningful clinical constructs. Notably, PID-5 trait scales have been found to be useful predictors of dropout from treatment completion, both in residential addiction treatment settings (Choate et al. 2021) and in intensive clinical settings for the treatment of personality disorders (Berghuis et al. 2021), further supporting the clinical usefulness of the instrument.

Another advantage of the AMPD is found in its integration of a developmental perspective in the assessment of personality-related pathology (De Clercq et al. 2009, 2014). Available literature suggests that personality disorders do not appear suddenly in adulthood, with an increasing amount of research indicating the importance of identifying emerging personality pathology in adolescence (e.g., De Fruyt and De Clercq 2014; Sharp 2017, 2020). The American Psychiatric Association released a version of the PID-5 for use with adolescents along with the version for adults, making available a measure of pathological personality domains and traits that can be used across different developmental periods. This release represents a fundamental step in assessing DSM-5 AMPD Criterion B in adolescence. Indeed, it should be observed that adopting a trait model in younger age groups is consistent with available evidence showing the continuities between childhood and adult dimensional trait models (e.g., Caspi et al. 2005; De Fruyt et al. 2006; Shiner et al. 2003). Adopting a dimensional perspective in conceptualizing personality pathology in adolescence may be useful in allowing for a fine-grained understanding of the developmental fluctuations and heterogeneity of personality disorder characteristics reported in younger samples (i.e., De Fruyt and De Clercq 2014), while avoiding potentially stigmatizing diagnostic jargon.

Notably, De Clercq et al. (2014) were the first authors to administer the PID-5 to a nonclinical sample of adolescents, finding support for its internal consistency reliability, factor structure, and convergent validity with age-specific facets of personality pathology. Further support for the reliability and validity of the PID-5 across different samples of adolescents and young adults was provided in subsequent studies (e.g., De Caluwé et al. 2019; Somma et al. 2017). Finally, the PID-5 proved useful in addressing relevant clinical outcomes in adolescence. For instance, Somma et al. (2016) carried out a study in an inpatient sample, which supported the usefulness of selected PID-5 traits (i.e., depressivity, anhedonia, and submissiveness) in profiling adolescents at risk for life-threatening suicide attempts. Moreover, the PID-5 Negative Affect score proved to be a significant predictor of clinicians' ratings of nonsuicidal self-injury severity in a sample of adolescent inpatients even when the effect of the depression was held constant, supporting the usefulness of the PID-5 in understanding risk factors for nonsuicidal self-injury (Somma et al. 2019a). A more detailed description of different versions of the PID-5 for use in adolescence is provided in Chapter 3, "The PID-5s."

CROSS-CULTURAL VALIDITY

The increasing popularity of the PID-5 in different countries and rapidly growing data on the PID-5 in both community and clinical samples stress the need for verifying cross-cultural generalizability of the measurement properties of the PID-5. By aiming for accurate assessment of the 25 traits and 5 domains constituting DSM-5 AMPD Criterion B, the PID-5 provides clinicians and their patients with reliable scores that validly represent core dimensions of dysfunctional personality that can be assessed meaningfully in the presence of human cultural diversity. In this respect, providing information on cross-cultural properties of the PID-5 became vital to clinical utility, acting as a necessary framework for integrating scientific findings from different countries and cultures.

The need for cross-cultural information on PID-5 psychometric properties prompted a burgeoning, spontaneously initiated worldwide research program. To appreciate the effectiveness of this research initiative, it should be considered that 3 years after the release of DSM-5, Al-Dajani et al. (2016) were already able to carry out the first systematic review of the psychometric properties of the PID-5, based on 39 independent samples from 30 published studies collected across different countries. After Al-Dajani et al.'s (2016) study was published, the body of research data on PID-5 psychometric properties across the world grew even faster. In turn, the availability of an impressive amount of research data allowed for meta-analyses of PID-5 factor structure, including data from multiple countries (Watters and Bagby 2018). Somma et al. (2019b) conducted the first meta-analysis of PID-5 factor structure, finding support for the reproducibility of the PID-5 domain factor structure in U.S. and non-U.S. cultural contexts. Finally, Barchi-Ferreira Bel and Osório (2020) carried out a second systematic review of the published literature on the PID-5, examining 64 additional studies with respect to Al-Dajani et al.'s (2016) review and including data on the short-form and informant-rated versions of the PID-5. Barchi-Ferreira Bel and Osório's (2020) systematic review aimed at providing information on the reliability, construct validity, and criterion-related validity of different versions of the PID-5 to show its suitability for use in different cultures and contexts.

What Have We Learned From Data on the PID-5 Psychometric Properties Across Different Cultures?

As a whole, systematic reviews (Al-Dajani et al. 2016; Barchi-Ferreira Bel and Osório 2020; Somma et al. 2019b; Watters and Bagby 2018) have suggested that the 220-item version of the PID-5 shows adequate internal consistency reliability estimates (i.e., Cronbach's α/McDonald's ω coefficient values >0.70) for both trait and domain scale scores in community and clinical samples, with apparent cross-cultural generalizability. Lower internal consistency reliabilities were reported only in non-U.S. studies and only for the Suspiciousness facet score. Adequate internal consistency reliability coefficient values were reported also for the short-form and informant-rated versions of the PID-5, although the amount of available data on these forms is relatively limited. Despite the relative sparseness of the scientific evidence on this topic, the PID-5 scale scores seem to demonstrate adequate test-retest reliability estimates over 2-week to 4-month time intervals in different countries.

The five-factor structure of the 220-item PID-5 trait scale scores has been consistently replicated across the United States and other countries, as well as across adult and adolescent samples and community and clinical samples. In different samples from different countries, the PID-5 scale scores showed meaningful, substantial, and significant associations with potentially adaptive personality dimensions (e.g., Five Factor Model trait measure scores). In terms of the criterion-related validity of PID-5 scale scores, the presence of significant, clinically relevant, and substantial correlations with measures of personality disorders is a consistently replicated finding from multiple studies from different cultures, countries, and populations (e.g., adult and adolescent samples, community-dwelling samples, clinical and forensic samples). The consistency of these correlational patterns across different studies, different samples, and different cultures led Watters et al. (2019) to carry out extensive meta-analytic research to provide empirically derived PID-5 dysfunctional profiles for the six personality disorder diagnoses retained in DSM-5 Section III (namely, antisocial, avoidant, borderline, narcissistic, obsessive-compulsive, and schizotypal personality disorders).

Thus, available evidence seems to indicate that the PID-5, especially in its 220-item version, can be used effectively to assess DSM-5 AMPD Criterion B dysfunctional personality dimensions in different cultures and contexts. These findings may have important implications for using PID-5 profiles for case conceptualization among clinicians from different cultures, as well as for integrating PID-5 research findings from different countries.

Future Directions

Notwithstanding these promising data, research is far from conclusive in supporting PID-5 cross-cultural validity. The PID-5 has been officially translated into only a relatively limited set of languages (e.g., Arabic, Chinese, Czech, Danish, Dutch, Farsi, French, German, Italian, Norwegian, Portuguese, Spanish, Swedish); more data on different linguistic and cultural contexts are needed before drawing firm conclusions. The number of available studies providing evidence for cross-cultural validity of the scale differs markedly across the different forms of the PID-5, thus preventing extension of knowledge on the 220-item version of the scale to other PID-5 forms. Long-term test-retest reliability information (i.e., test-retest intervals of 1 year or longer) is still unavailable for all versions of the PID-5 in its different translations.

PID-5 AS A TOOL FOR UNDERSTANDING DIVERSITY

The consistency of the PID-5 psychometric properties across different languages and countries seems to support its potential usefulness in multicultural populations such as in the United States. However, Bagby et al. (2022) examined the factor structure of the PID-5 in two racial groups within the United States (White Americans and Black Americans) and found a lack of configural invariance (i.e., equivalence of model form) across the two groups. Although Bagby et al. (2022) found that the expected five-factor structure fit best among White Americans, a single-factor structure reflecting general demoralization fit best among Black Americans. Nevertheless, in an attempt to replicate these findings, Freilich et al. (2023) carried out follow-up analyses in an independent sample of 613 Black Americans and 612 White Americans and found support for strong measurement invariance across the two groups. Although replication is needed, Freilich et al.'s (2023) findings suggest that PID-5 trait and domain observed scores between White American and Black American groups can be compared appropriately.

In line with cross-cultural data supporting the clinical usefulness of the PID-5 in different cultures and contexts, Maples-Keller et al. (2021) supported the use of the 25-item version of the PID-5 as a tool for assessing dysfunctional personality traits in highly traumatized African American women. Along the same lines, Becker et al. (2023) administered the 25-item version of the PID-5 in a large sample of partial hospital patients and found support for strong measurement invariance of the PID-5 factor structure between White and non-White groups. The PID-5 also has been shown to have utility in assessment among sexual minorities (e.g., Rodriguez-Seijas et al. 2021; Russell et al. 2017). For instance, Rodriguez-Seijas et al. (2021) relied on the 25-item version of the PID-5 to examine the nature of differences in prevalence of borderline personality disorder among sexual and gender minority individuals.

Of course, further studies on structural and psychometric generalizability of the PID-5 across different U.S. ethnic groups are needed. Moreover, understanding race and culture and investigating construct equivalence of the PID-5 trait and domain constructs across populations are important topics for current and future research (Bagby et al. 2022; Freilich et al. 2023). Despite encouraging findings, more work is needed to explore the psychometric properties and clinical utility of the PID-5 to assess dysfunctional personality traits in marginalized and minority groups.

REFERENCES

Al-Dajani N, Gralnick TM, Bagby RM: A psychometric review of the Personality Inventory for DSM-5 (PID-5): current status and future directions. J Pers Assess 98(1):62–81, 2016 26619968

American Psychiatric Association: Diagnostic and Statistical Manual of Mental Disorders, 4th Edition. Washington, DC, American Psychiatric Association, 1994

American Psychiatric Association: Diagnostic and Statistical Manual of Mental Disorders, 5th Edition. Washington, DC, American Psychiatric Association, 2013

Bagby RM, Keeley JW, Williams CC, et al: Evaluating the measurement invariance of the Personality Inventory for DSM-5 (PID-5) in Black Americans and white Americans. Psychol Assess 34(1):82–90, 2022 34871023

Barchi-Ferreira Bel AM, Osório FL: The Personality Inventory for DSM-5: psychometric evidence of validity and reliability—updates. Harv Rev Psychiatry 28(4):225–237, 2020 32692087

Becker LG, Asadi S, Zimmerman M, et al: Is there a bias in the diagnosis of borderline personality disorder among racially minoritized patients? Personal Disord 14(3):339–346, 2023 35549499

Berghuis H, Bandell CC, Krueger RF: Predicting dropout using DSM-5 Section II personality disorders, and DSM-5 Section III personality traits, in a (day)clinical sample of personality disorders. Pers Disord 12(4):331–338, 2021 32730060

Caspi A, Roberts BW, Shiner RL: Personality development: stability and change. Annu Rev Psychol 56:453–484, 2005 15709943

Choate AM, Gorey C, Rappaport LM, et al: Alternative model of personality disorders traits predict residential addictions treatment completion. Drug Alcohol Depend 228:109011, 2021 34521057

De Caluwé E, Verbeke L, Aken MV, et al: The DSM-5 trait measure in a psychiatric sample of late adolescents and emerging adults: structure, reliability, and validity. J Pers Disord 33(1):101–118, 2019 29469666

De Clercq B, De Fruyt F, Widiger TA: Integrating a developmental perspective in dimensional models of personality disorders. Clin Psychol Rev 29(2):154–162, 2009 19167138

De Clercq B, De Fruyt F, De Bolle M, et al: The hierarchical structure and construct validity of the PID-5 trait measure in adolescence. J Pers 82(2):158–169, 2014 23647646

De Fruyt F, De Clercq B: Antecedents of personality disorder in childhood and adolescence: toward an integrative developmental model. Annu Rev Clin Psychol 10:449–476, 2014 24471374

De Fruyt F, Bartels M, Van Leeuwen KG, et al: Five types of personality continuity in childhood and adolescence. J Pers Soc Psychol 91(3):538–552, 2006 16938036

Dunne AL, Gilbert F, Daffern M: Investigating the relationship between DSM-5 personality disorder domains and facets and aggression in an offender population using the Personality Inventory for the DSM-5. J Pers Disord 32(5):668–693, 2018 28972816

Few LR, Miller JD, Rothbaum AO, et al: Examination of the Section III DSM-5 diagnostic system for personality disorders in an outpatient clinical sample. J Abnorm Psychol 122(4):1057–1069, 2013 24364607

Freilich CD, Palumbo IM, Latzman RD, et al: Assessing the measurement invariance of the Personality Inventory for DSM-5 across Black and White Americans. Psychol Assess 35(9):721–728, 2023 37384515

Gore WL, Widiger TA: The DSM-5 dimensional trait model and five-factor models of general personality. J Abnorm Psychol 122(3):816–821, 2013 23815395

Hopwood CJ, Thomas KM, Markon KE, et al: DSM-5 personality traits and DSM-IV personality disorders. J Abnorm Psychol 121(2):424–432, 2012 22250660

Krueger RF, Derringer J, Markon KE, et al: Initial construction of a maladaptive personality trait model and inventory for DSM-5 [Erratum appears in Psychol Med 42(9):1891, 2012]. Psychol Med 42(9):1879–1890, 2012 22153017

Maples-Keller JL, Hyatt CS, Sleep CE, et al: DSM-5 alternative model for personality disorders trait domains and PTSD symptoms in a sample of highly traumatized African American women and a prospective sample of trauma center patients. Pers Disord 12(6):491–502, 2021 33444034

Quilty LC, Ayearst L, Chmielewski M, et al: The psychometric properties of the Personality Inventory for DSM-5 in an APA DSM-5 field trial sample. Assessment 20(3):362–369, 2013 23588687

Rodriguez-Seijas C, Morgan TA, Zimmerman M: Is there a bias in the diagnosis of borderline personality disorder among lesbian, gay, and bisexual patients? Assessment 28(3):724–738, 2021 32981328

Russell TD, Pocknell V, King AR: Lesbians and bisexual women and men have higher scores on the Personality Inventory for the DSM-5 (PID-5) than heterosexual counterparts. Pers Individ Dif 110:119–124, 2017

Sharp C: Bridging the gap: the assessment and treatment of adolescent personality disorder in routine clinical care. Arch Dis Child 102(1):103–108, 2017 27507846

Sharp C: Adolescent personality pathology and the alternative model for personality disorders: self development as nexus. Psychopathology 53(3–4):198–204, 2020 32464626

Shiner RL, Masten AS, Roberts JM: Childhood personality foreshadows adult personality and life outcomes two decades later. J Pers 71(6):1145–1170, 2003 14633061

Somma A, Fossati A, Terrinoni A, et al: Reliability and clinical usefulness of the Personality Inventory for DSM-5 in clinically referred adolescents: a preliminary report in a sample of Italian inpatients. Compr Psychiatry 70:141–151, 2016 27624434

Somma A, Borroni S, Maffei C, et al: Reliability, factor structure, and associations with measures of problem relationship and behavior of the Personality Inventory for DSM-5 in a sample of Italian community-dwelling adolescents. J Pers Disord 31(5):624–646, 2017 28072038

Somma A, Fossati A, Ferrara M, et al: DSM-5 personality domains as correlates of non-suicidal self-injury severity in an Italian sample of adolescent inpatients with self-destructive behaviour. Pers Ment Health 13(4):205–214, 2019a 31353830

Somma A, Krueger RF, Markon KE, et al: The replicability of the Personality Inventory for DSM-5 domain scale factor structure in U.S. and non-U.S. samples: a quantitative review of the published literature. Psychol Assess 31(7):861–877, 2019b 30883152

Watters CA, Bagby RM: A meta-analysis of the five-factor internal structure of the Personality Inventory for DSM-5. Psychol Assess 30(9):1255–1260, 2018 29952594

Watters CA, Bagby RM, Sellbom M: Meta-analysis to derive an empirically based set of personality facet criteria for the alternative DSM-5 model for personality disorders. Pers Disord 10(2):97–104, 2019 30520649

Wright AGC, Calabrese WR, Rudick MM, et al: Stability of the DSM-5 Section III pathological personality traits and their longitudinal associations with psychosocial functioning in personality disordered individuals. J Abnorm Psychol 124(1):199–207, 2015 25384070

CHAPTER 3

The PID-5s

DIFFERENT VERSIONS FOR DIFFERENT NEEDS

Although most research on the Personality Inventory for DSM-5 (PID-5; American Psychiatric Association 2013) has relied on the 220-item version, researchers and clinicians may choose among different versions of the PID-5 depending on their assessment needs and available time. In 2013, the American Psychiatric Association released three different versions of the PID-5 for adults: the 220-item self-report version, a 25-item version, and a 218-item informant-report version. They also made available two forms of the PID-5 for use with adolescents ages 11–17 years, which include the same items as the corresponding adult forms: the 220-item self-report version and the 25-item version. From this perspective, the PID-5 has comprised a family of instruments since the beginning.

After the official release of the DSM-5 Online Assessment Measures, other versions of the PID-5 were developed by researchers working in the field of personality assessment. In this chapter, different versions of the PID-5 that are designed to assess DSM-5 dysfunctional personality traits and domains are discussed. (Specific forms of the PID-5 that are designed to target specific clinical needs, such as the assessment of psychopathy or the promotion of communication between different diagnostic systems, are discussed in Chapter 5, "Special Applications of the PID-5.") Table 3–1 summarizes the main characteristics of the different versions of the PID-5. Researchers and clinicians may select the

Table 3–1. Main characteristics of the different versions of the Personality Inventory for DSM-5 (PID-5)

Version	Items	Age group	Time to complete	Trait and domain scales	Validity scales
PID-5	220 items, self-report	Adults and adolescents[a]	20–25 min	25 trait scales 5 domain scales	3 scales: Inconsistent responding Overreporting Underreporting
PID-5-SF	100 items, self-report	Adults and adolescents[a]	10–15 min	25 trait scales 5 domain scales	1 scale: Inconsistent responding
PD-5-BF	25 items, self-report	Adults and adolescents[a]	5–10 min	5 domain scales 1 total score (domain profile elevation)	
PID-5-IRF	218 items, informant report	Adults	20–25 min	25 trait scales 5 domain scales	

Note.   BF=Brief Form; IRF=Informant Form; SF=Short Form.
[a] Adolescent norms are currently unavailable in the United States; further research is needed on use of the PID-5 with adolescents in the United States.

most appropriate version of the measure depending on their assessment needs (e.g., evaluating dysfunctional personality traits requires longer versions of the instrument), resources (e.g., time), and assessment setting (e.g., psychiatric, medical, legal, educational, psychological clinic setting).

PERSONALITY INVENTORY FOR DSM-5—BRIEF FORM

General Description

The Personality Inventory for DSM-5—Brief Form (PID-5-BF) is a 25-item self-report form released by the American Psychiatric Association. The PID-5-BF items come from the 220-item self-report PID-5, and they map content from the most strongly loading facets identified in the PID-5, representing 21 of the 25 PID-5 trait facets. As in the PID-5, each PID-5-BF item is rated on a 4-point scale, ranging from "0=very false or often false" to "3=very true or often true," and each PID-5-BF item is scored on only one PID-5-BF domain scale. The PID-5-BF was designed to assess the five DSM-5 Alternative Model for Personality Disorders (AMPD) dysfunctional domains of negative affectivity, detachment, antagonism, disinhibition, and psychoticism, with each domain scale consisting of five items. Unlike the other versions of the PID-5, the PID-5-BF total score can be computed by averaging the overall score by the total number of items in the measure (i.e., 25). It is notable that the PID-5-BF was not designed as a fine-grained measure for assessing AMPD traits; rather, it was meant to screen for possible personality pathology and to assess AMPD dysfunctional personality domains when time and resources are limited. With this aim in mind, researchers and clinicians can consider the PID-5-BF total score in situations in which quantifying the overall level of personality psychopathology is a concern.

Available data show that the PID-5-BF scores show adequate psychometric properties in undergraduate, community, psychiatric, primary care clinic, and forensic adult samples (Anderson et al. 2018; Bach et al. 2016; Dunne et al. 2021; Gomez et al. 2020; Porcerelli et al. 2019), with acceptable to excellent internal consistency reliability and factor validity. Moreover, the PID-5-BF showed adequate convergent validity with the 220-item version of the PID-5 domains and adaptive and maladaptive personality measures (e.g., Anderson et al. 2018; Bach et al. 2016). Additionally, PID-5-BF criterion validity with respect to DSM-5

Section II personality disorder diagnoses and internalizing and externalizing psychopathology has been confirmed (e.g., Anderson et al. 2018; Bach et al. 2016). Accordingly, the PID-5-BF could represent a sound and clinically useful screening measure of maladaptive personality (e.g., Anderson et al. 2018).

Even though the PID-5-BF was designed as a self-report measure, its positive features (e.g., brevity) point to other possible applications, such as adaptations as a brief informant form. For example, in a large study that was designed to assess dysfunctional personality traits in clinical youths, the parents were asked to complete the 25 items of the PID-5-BF to briefly describe their children's personality (Koster et al. 2022).

Use in Adolescents

Although current unavailability of norms precludes its clinical use with adolescents in the United States at this time, research in other countries suggests that the PID-5-BF can be administered to both adults and adolescents ages 11–17 years. The availability and routine use of a brief screen for personality pathology could potentially allow for the earlier detection of personality disorders in adolescents. From this point of view, use of the PID-5-BF could increase the likelihood that practitioners alerted to the possibility of personality pathology would pursue a more formal evaluation of possible personality problems (e.g., Noblin et al. 2014).

Interestingly, support was found for PID-5-BF internal consistency, 2-month test-retest reliability, factor structure, and associations with a measure of personality functioning in adolescents (Fossati et al. 2017). Recently, the PID-5-BF was shown to be useful in screening for borderline personality disorder in college students (Cano et al. 2022).

PERSONALITY INVENTORY FOR DSM-5—SHORT FORM

General Description

The Personality Inventory for DSM-5—Short Form (PID-5-SF) is a 100-item self-report form developed after the release of the PID-5. PID-5-SF items were selected from the 220-item version of the PID-5, relying on item response theory methods (Maples et al. 2015). Four items per scale were chosen to provide adequate content coverage of the traits along with maximum measurement precision. The scoring algorithm for the PID-5-SF items was provided by Maples et al. (2015, appendix) and is summarized in Table 3–2.

Table 3–2. Personality Inventory for DSM-5—Short Form (PID-5-SF) items

PID-5-SF trait scale	PID-5 item numbers
Anxiousness	79, 109, 130, 174
Emotional lability	122, 138, 165, 181
Hostility	38, 92, 158, 170
Perseveration	60, 80, 100, 128
(Lack of) restricted affectivity	84,[a] 91,[a] 167,[a] 184[a]
Separation insecurity	50, 127, 149, 175
Submissiveness	9, 15, 63, 202
Anhedonia	23, 26, 124, 157
Depressivity	81, 151, 163, 169
Intimacy avoidance	89, 120, 145, 203
Suspiciousness	2, 117, 133, 190
Withdrawal	82, 136, 146, 186
Attention seeking	74, 173, 191, 211
Callousness	19, 153, 166, 183
Deceitfulness	53, 134, 206, 218
Grandiosity	40, 114, 187, 197
Manipulativeness	107, 125, 162, 219
Distractibility	118, 132, 144, 199
Impulsivity	4, 16, 17, 22
Irresponsibility	129, 156, 160, 171
(Lack of) rigid perfectionism	105,[a] 123,[a] 176,[a] 196[a]
Risk taking	39, 48, 67, 159
Eccentricity	25, 70, 152, 205
Perceptual dysregulation	44, 154, 192, 217
Unusual beliefs and experiences	106, 139, 150, 209

[a]Reverse-scored item.

The PID-5-SF is a subset of the full PID-5, and as with the PID-5, each item is rated on a 4-point scale, ranging from "0=very false or often false" to "3=very true or often true." Also in line with the full-length version of the PID-5, the PID-5-SF enables clinicians and researchers to assess the five AMPD dysfunctional domains of negative affectivity, detachment, antagonism, disinhibition, and psychoticism and the 25 specific personality traits. Maples and colleagues (2015) showed that the PID-5 trait and domain scales have similar reliability, factor structure, and correlational properties as the 220-item version of the PID-5 in general and clinical populations.

Since the publication of the PID-5-SF (Maples et al. 2015), additional studies have demonstrated the instrument's psychometric properties and clinical utility. For instance, the PID-5-SF trait scale five-factor structure replicated the internal structure of the original PID-5 in Danish community and clinical samples (Bach et al. 2016). In addition, Thimm et al. (2016) showed that the Norwegian PID-5-SF was a reliable and efficient measure of the trait criterion of the AMPD in a sample of university students. Finally, Somma et al. (2019) showed that the use of the PID-5-SF did not result in a substantial loss of information as compared with the original PID-5 in either general or clinical population samples. In summary, the PID-5-SF provides an excellent compromise between comprehensiveness and the time required for completion of the measure.

Use in Adolescents

The PID-5-SF has been shown to be a reliable and efficient measure of the DSM-5 dysfunctional personality traits and domains in adolescents (e.g., See et al. 2020). Koster et al. (2020) provided further evidence for extended applicability of the PID-5-SF for both clinical and nonclinical populations of mid- and late adolescents. Because of its positive psychometric features and its clinical utility, the PID-5-SF was recently selected as a measure of dispositional traits in a longitudinal research project aimed at studying maladaptive personality development in clinical youths between 12 and 24 years (Koster et al. 2022).

PERSONALITY INVENTORY FOR DSM-5—INFORMANT FORM

The Personality Inventory for DSM-5—Informant Form (PID-5-IRF) is the informant version of the PID-5 released by the American Psychiatric

Association; it comprises 218 informant-rated items and allows dysfunctional personality trait and domain assessment for adults ages 18 and older. This measure is particularly useful for those situations in which gathering collateral information on the patient is helpful or necessary. The PID-5-IRF was developed to be completed by an adult informant responding about another individual they know well. Specifically, each item asks the informant to rate how well the item describes the individual generally.

As in the PID-5, each PID-5-IRF item is rated on a 4-point scale, ranging from "0=very false or often false" to "3=very true or often true." This measure has 25 primary scales that correspond to the dysfunctional personality traits in the AMPD, along with the 5 higher-order domain scales: negative affectivity, detachment, antagonism, disinhibition, and psychoticism.

The PID-5-IRF has been shown to be a useful measure for several scenarios (e.g., when additional sources of information are desired, when informant measures are expected to provide incremental validity over self-report, when relationships or social perception is a focal interest, or when response bias is a salient concern) (Markon et al. 2013). Its use has not necessarily been limited to friends or family of patients; for example, the PID-5-IRF was used as a systematic measure of dimensional traits to assess agreement between therapists and patients, showing that therapists' agreement with patients was higher than reported in previous studies (Samuel et al. 2018).

SELECTING THE OPTIMAL VERSION OF THE PID-5 FOR SPECIFIC ASSESSMENT SITUATIONS

As detailed in the previous paragraph, different assessment situations may require clinicians and researchers to select the most appropriate version of the PID-5. Figure 3–1 presents a decision tree designed to help assessors in identifying the most appropriate version of the PID-5, depending on time restrictions and clinical needs.

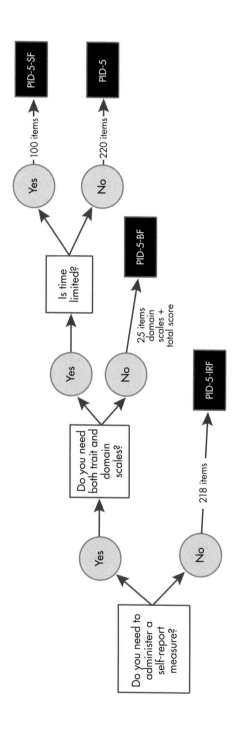

Figure 3–1. Decision tree for choosing the most appropriate Personality Inventory for DSM-5 (PID-5) version.

BF=Brief Form; IRF=Informant Form; SF=Short Form.

REFERENCES

American Psychiatric Association: Diagnostic and Statistical Manual of Mental Disorders, 5th Edition. Washington, DC, American Psychiatric Association, 2013

Anderson JL, Sellbom M, Salekin RT: Utility of the Personality Inventory for DSM-5–Brief Form (PID-5-BF) in the measurement of maladaptive personality and psychopathology. Assessment 25(5):596–607, 2018 27827808

Bach B, Maples-Keller JL, Bo S, et al: The alternative DSM-5 personality disorder traits criterion: a comparative examination of three self-report forms in a Danish population. Personal Disord 7(2):124–135, 2016 26642229

Cano K, Sumlin E, Sharp C: Screening for borderline personality pathology on college campuses. Pers Ment Health 16(3):235–243, 2022 34910370

Dunne AL, Trounson JS, Skues J, et al: The Personality Inventory for DSM-5–Brief Form: an examination of internal consistency, factor structure, and relationship to aggression in an incarcerated offender sample. Assessment 28(4):1136–1146, 2021 33563023

Fossati A, Somma A, Borroni S, et al: The Personality Inventory for DSM-5 Brief Form: evidence for reliability and construct validity in a sample of community-dwelling Italian adolescents. Assessment 24(5):615–631, 2017 26676917

Gomez R, Watson S, Stavropoulos V: Personality Inventory for DSM-5, Brief Form: factor structure, reliability, and coefficient of congruence. Personal Disord 11(1):69–77, 2020 31670543

Koster N, Laceulle OM, Van der Heijden PT, et al: A psychometric evaluation of a reduced version of the PID-5 in clinical and nonclinical adolescents. Eur J Psychol Assess 36:758–766, 2020

Koster N, Lusin I, van der Heijden PT, et al: Understanding personality pathology in a clinical sample of youth: study protocol for the longitudinal research project "APOLO." BMJ Open 12(6):e054485, 2022 35732393

Maples JL, Carter NT, Few LR, et al: Testing whether the DSM-5 personality disorder trait model can be measured with a reduced set of items: an item response theory investigation of the Personality Inventory for DSM-5. Psychol Assess 27(4):1195–1210, 2015 25844534

Markon KE, Quilty LC, Bagby RM, et al: The development and psychometric properties of an informant-report form of the Personality Inventory for DSM-5 (PID-5). Assessment 20(3):370–383, 2013 23612961

Noblin JL, Venta A, Sharp C: The validity of the MSI-BPD among inpatient adolescents. Assessment 21(2):210–217, 2014 23344914

Porcerelli JH, Hopwood CJ, Jones JR: Convergent and discriminant validity of Personality Inventory for DSM-5-BF in a primary care sample. J Pers Disord 33(6):846–856, 2019 30355021

Samuel DB, Suzuki T, Bucher MA, et al: The agreement between clients' and their therapists' ratings of personality disorder traits. J Consult Clin Psychol 86(6):546–555, 2018 29781652

See AY, Klimstra TA, Cramer AOJ, et al: The network structure of personality pathology in adolescence with the 100-item Personality Inventory for DSM-5 Short-Form (PID-5-SF). Front Psychol 11:823, 2020 32431646

Somma A, Krueger RF, Markon KE, et al: Item response theory analyses, factor structure, and external correlates of the Italian translation of the Personality Inventory for DSM-5 Short Form in community-dwelling adults and clinical adults. Assessment 26(5):839–852, 2019 29902930

Thimm JC, Jordan S, Bach B: The Personality Inventory for DSM-5 Short Form (PID-5-SF): psychometric properties and association with big five traits and pathological beliefs in a Norwegian population. BMC Psychol 4(1):61, 2016 27927237

CHAPTER 4

PID-5 Response Validity Assessment and Validity Scales

The reliability, validity, and clinical utility of the Personality Inventory for DSM-5 (PID-5; American Psychiatric Association 2013) in diverse cultural contexts and languages have been extensively documented (see Chapter 2, "Basic Measurement Properties and Validity of the PID-5 Across Populations"). However, validity scales were suggested early as a possible necessity for use of the PID-5 in some contexts, such as forensic settings (see, e.g., McGee Ng et al. 2016). When individuals respond to test items noncredibly, the interpretability of the results may be diminished or compromised. This may complicate the interpretability of PID-5 profiles, especially when clinicians rely solely on self-report versions of the PID-5 for the assessment of dysfunctional personality traits and domains.

To address these concerns, researchers have developed embedded validity scales for the PID-5 to provide an efficient assessment of threats to interpretability of the validity of PID-5 protocols. In general, PID-5 validity scales assess three types of threats to the interpretability of test scores: response inconsistency, overreporting, and underreporting. In this chapter, the logic behind the development of PID-5 validity scales is detailed, including scoring and guidelines for interpretation.

INCONSISTENT AND INCOHERENT RESPONDING

Response inconsistency occurs when a respondent does not attend to or understand the PID-5 items or otherwise responds incoherently to them. Previous data have shown that inattentive response can be common; estimated rates of inattention have varied significantly across studies on the basis of the definition of the construct. Some studies have reported rates ranging from 3% to 46% of respondents (Meade and Craig 2012), with estimates of 10%–12% of students answering superficially to questionnaires (e.g., Maniaci and Rogge 2014; Meade and Craig 2012).

In clinical contexts, failing to identify inconsistent responses may lead to inappropriate interpretation of test results. For example, if random answers artificially produce high scores on psychopathology scales (Keeley et al. 2016), identification of treatment targets may be distorted. We can imagine a situation in which the score on PID-5 Anxiousness, measuring feelings of nervousness, tenseness, or panic in reaction to various situations, may not be representative of the subject's real position on that specific dimension. This may lead to an erroneous focus on mechanisms associated with neuroticism during treatment planning. Similar considerations hold for research and other large-scale assessment contexts, in which inattentive responses may affect reliability and correlations between PID-5 measures and criterion variables (e.g., Curran 2016).

Inconsistent responding may be related to several factors, such as inattention, fatigue, confusion, noncooperation, or comprehension difficulties. Moreover, some studies (e.g., Bowling et al. 2016) have suggested that inattention during testing can be relatively stable across time and situations, raising the possibility that if observed, inconsistency might recur. Accordingly, clinicians and researchers need to carefully assess possible reasons for inconsistent responding and consider the implications of different strategies for addressing response invalidity on a case-by-case basis.

Variable Response Inconsistency Scale for PID-5

In order to address concerns related to random responding, Keeley and colleagues (2016) proposed a scale to detect inconsistency in PID-5 responses, the PID-5 Variable Response Inconsistency (VRIN) validity scale. The procedure in developing this scale was similar to that used in developing the Minnesota Multiphasic Personality Inventory (MMPI) VRIN scale (e.g., Butcher et al. 2001).

Keeley and colleagues (2016) first identified 41 highly associated PID-5 item pairs (correlating more than 0.60) and then examined their content to determine whether they were sufficiently similar. Redundant item pairs were then removed. Finally, highly correlated pairs of PID-5 items having similar content and coming from the same PID-5 trait scale were included in the final inconsistency scale. PID-5-VRIN items were selected so as to have 1) similar content, 2) maximum correlation within the pairs, and 3) minimum values of correlations between pairs (Keeley et al. 2016). This process resulted in the identification of 20 pairs of items, which constitute the PID-5-VRIN scale.

The item pairs included in the PID-5-VRIN are listed in Table 4–1. An inconsistency score is calculated by summing the absolute values of the differences between the participant's raw answers for each set of paired items (Keeley et al. 2016). Because PID-5-VRIN item differences can range from 0 (perfect consistency) to 3 (perfect inconsistency) for each pair of PID-5 items, the possible total PID-5-VRIN score ranges from 0 to 60.

Keeley and colleagues (2016) documented that the VRIN scale was able to reliably distinguish genuine answers from random answers for both college students and respondents in clinical samples and proposed a cutoff score of 17 or greater to indicate an invalid PID-5 profile. The utility of this PID-5-VRIN cutoff also was confirmed in general population, clinical, and adolescent samples in a different (Italian) cultural context (Somma et al. 2018), suggesting that the PID-5-VRIN scale is useful for assessing response inconsistency on the PID-5.

In the U.S. normative sample, the mean PID-5-VRIN score was 8.16 and the median score was 8, with an SD of 4.69. Given this, a cutoff of 17 would correspond to a z score of 1.88 and the 96th percentile of PID-5-VRIN scores. Replicating the procedure of randomly replacing half of the individuals' response patterns in the normative sample with random responses and repeating this process suggests that accuracy of classification is maximized at a PID-5-VRIN score of 15, at which overall accuracy in identifying a response pattern as genuine or random is approximately 94%. The overall accuracy of a cutoff of 17 in the normative sample when using this process is lower, approximately 91%. Given the replicated cutoff of 17 in other studies and types of samples, however, and because it is more conservative, we recommend using a cutoff of 17, although scores in the range of 15–17 might be considered for further investigation depending on the setting.

When test takers obtain scores higher than or equal to 17 on the PID-5-VRIN, the PID-5 trait and domain profile should be interpreted with

Table 4–1. Personality Inventory for DSM-5 Variable Response Inconsistency (PID-5-VRIN) scale/PID-5—Short Form Response Inconsistency Scale (PID-5-INC-S) item pairs

PID-5 scales	PID-5-VRIN item pairs[a]
Anxiousness	79-174[b]
Anxiousness	109-110
Emotional lability	102-122
Emotional lability	138-181[b]
Hostility	38-92
Perseveration	80-128[b]
Separation insecurity	50-127[b]
Depressivity	148-169[b]
Intimacy avoidance	89-145[b]
Attention seeking	74-173[b]
Attention seeking	191-211[b]
Callousness	153-166[b]
Manipulativeness	125-180
Rigid perfectionism	105-123[b]
Distractibility	132-144
Eccentricity	21-55
Eccentricity	24-25
Eccentricity	52-152
Eccentricity	70-71
Eccentricity	172-185

[a]PID-5 item numbers refer to the 220-item version of the instrument.
[b]Item pairs included in the PID-5-INC-S.

caution because the test results may be inaccurate. Of course, PID-5-VRIN scores higher than or equal to 17 do not necessarily imply that the test taker was intentionally uncooperative or otherwise responding randomly. Indeed, as mentioned earlier, invalid PID-5 protocols may be the result of the different processes and should be investigated by the assessor by examining collateral and other information (e.g., the respondent's attitude toward testing, time spent on the test, moment of the day, knowledge of the language). Notably, it should be observed that the same PID-5-VRIN score may be associated with different potential causes.

Under certain circumstances (e.g., if the person was particularly tired when completing the questionnaire), assessors may have reason to believe that the examinee may provide more accurate responses if the test is readministered. Of course, this judgment is related to the context (e.g., clinical vs. forensic settings), characteristics of the patient (adolescent vs. adult), and reasons for not being able to complete the PID-5 in a consistent manner (inattentiveness vs. low motivation).

PID-5—Short Form Response Inconsistency Scale

Lowmaster et al. (2020) developed a response inconsistency scale for the 100-item version of the PID-5, the PID-5—Short Form (PID-5-SF; Maples et al. 2015). Building on Keeley et al.'s (2016) work, Lowmaster et al. (2020, 2021) considered 10-item pairs included in both the 220-item version and the 100-item version of the PID-5 and evaluated whether they could be effective in detecting inconsistent responding on the PID-5-SF. Across three independent studies, Lowmaster et al. (2020) developed and cross-validated the PID-5-SF Response Inconsistency Scale (PID-5-INC-S), showing that its scores were useful in discriminating randomly generated from real PID-5-SF protocols.

The items included in the PID-5-INC-S are listed in Table 4–1, indicated by superscript b. In line with the computation of the PID-5-VRIN, the PID-5-INC-S total score is calculated by summing the absolute differences of the 10 PID-5-SF item pairs; thus, the PID-5-INC-S total score can range from 0 to 30. Lowmaster et al. (2020, 2021) suggested a cutoff score of 8 or higher for accurately identifying inconsistent responses on the PID-5-SF.

Infrequency Items

Two items intended to mark inconsistent or incoherent responding were included in the normative data collection: "Every day, I forget my own name more than once" and "Every day, I forget where I was born more than once." With regard to these statements, 94% and 96% of individuals, respectively, responded "very false"; 3% and 2% responded "somewhat false," and 2% and 1% responded "somewhat true." No individuals in the normative sample endorsed "very true" to either. Only 1% of individuals endorsed both items simultaneously to some extent (i.e., responded "very true" or "somewhat true" to both). When coded in the direction of endorsement, the sum of these two items was correlated 0.25 with the PID-5-VRIN scale.

Given the nature of these two items, their extreme response distribution, and the relationship with the PID-5-VRIN scale, it seems reasonable to use these items as a screen for inconsistent or incoherent responding. Profiles from individuals who endorse one or both of these items should be interpreted with caution, and further inquiry into their responses is warranted. Such responses may reflect inconsistent or incoherent responding; it is also possible that individuals with such responses are systematically presenting themselves as implausibly cognitively impaired, suggesting the possibility of impression management, somatic symptom disorders, or other issues.

RESPONSE BIAS AND IMPRESSION MANAGEMENT

In contrast to inconsistent responding, in which respondents answer in a way that appears random, variable, or otherwise inconsistent, other individuals may answer systematically in a way that is biased relative to a "true" or consensus representation of their personality and functioning. In such cases, an individual may, for whatever reason, systematically overreport or underreport their level of psychopathology, leading to a distorted representation of their functioning on a psychological measure. More generally, response biases can be thought of in terms of factors systematically influencing the test responses other than the traits of interest, especially when those factors are induced by the measurement process itself.

Negative Impression Management and Overreported Psychopathology

Negative Impression Management

Across different assessment contexts, some individuals may be motivated to or have an incentive to exaggerate, fabricate, or otherwise overreport personality psychopathology (Rogers and Bender 2018). Overreporting or negative impression management refers to an unexpectedly high level of endorsement of items indicating psychopathology given an individual's actual level of psychopathology. Overreporting may be suspected when respondents present with a degree of dysfunction that seems noncredible (e.g., endorsement of items that seems excessive in severity or frequency). It may reflect any one or more of various factors, such as truly severe psychopathology, the presence of significant medical conditions, intentional response distortion, malingering, or desperation in seeking help. Moreover, exaggeration of personality psychopathology may be unintentional; for example, individuals with anxiety or depressive disorder may perceive and report their dysfunctional personality traits as more severe or impairing than they actually are. Similar considerations hold for people who are used to providing overemphatic descriptions of events and situations (e.g., Bagby et al. 2008).

Of course, negative impression management cannot be inferred by examining PID-5 scores alone. The assessment of overreporting and possible reasons for doing so, including intentionality, motivations, and internal or external incentives, should be based on careful consideration of collateral and other available information.

Assessment of overreporting and inaccurate reporting of personality dysfunction is relevant across a wide range of contexts (e.g., Rogers and Bender 2018). Although the phenomenon of negative impression management has been discussed widely in the forensic literature because individuals being evaluated in those settings may be highly motivated to simulate psychopathology, this occurs in other clinical and research settings as well. Several studies have found that an overreporting style may undermine scale accuracy and validity in both psychopathology and personality assessments (e.g., Burchett and Bagby 2014; Burchett and Ben-Porath 2010; Sellbom and Bagby 2008). These considerations underscore the need to assess overreporting of psychopathological symptoms in the context of clinical assessment (e.g., Al-Dajani et al. 2016).

PID-5 Over-Reporting Scale

Recognizing the importance of overreporting as a source of score distortion, Sellbom et al. (2018) developed a scale to detect overreporting on the PID-5. The PID-5 Over-Reporting Scale (PID-5-ORS) is a validity scale embedded in the 220-item self-report version of the measure.

In developing the PID-5-ORS, Sellbom et al. (2018) considered a rare symptom approach previously used in developing MMPI validity scales. Specifically, Sellbom et al. (2018) identified PID-5 items that rarely (≤5%) received an extreme response option (i.e., "very true or often true") across three independent student samples and a clinical outpatient sample. A total of 28 items were initially selected on the basis of this criterion; subsequently, for each PID-5 domain, the 2 items that were the least frequently endorsed were selected. To avoid content overlap, no PID-5 trait scale could contain more than one of the selected infrequently endorsed items. This process resulted in the identification of 10 PID-5 items.

The PID-5 item pairs selected to be included in the PID-5-ORS are listed in Table 4–2. To compute the PID-5-ORS total score, PID-5 users must first recode the PID-5-ORS item responses as either 0 or 1, where 1 reflects the most extreme response option ("very true or often true") and 0 reflects any other response. The PID-5-ORS is equal to the sum of these recoded responses.

The PID-5-ORS includes 10 items; accordingly, the PID-5-ORS total score ranges from 0 to a maximum of 10. The PID-5-ORS has shown adequate internal consistency reliability and moderate and significant associations with different well-established scales assessing overreporting style (e.g., the MMPI-2-Restructured Form overreporting validity scales). Notably, Sellbom et al. (2018) suggested an ideal cutoff score of 3 for optimally detecting possible overreporting of psychopathology on the PID-5. In the U.S. normative sample, scores on the PID-5-ORS were highly positively skewed, with 91% of respondents scoring 0 on this scale and 99% scoring less than the recommended cutoff of 3.

When respondents obtain scores of 3 or greater on the PID-5-ORS, they may have provided noncredible responses. As Sellbom et al. (2018) pointed out, the PID-5-ORS scores should be interpreted after ruling out inconsistent responding. Because the development of the PID-5-ORS was based on a rare symptom strategy, PID-5 overreporting indicators are highly susceptible to random, careless, or otherwise inconsistent responding. In the normative sample, for example, PID-5-VRIN scale and PID-5-ORS scores were correlated 0.22.

If inconsistent responding is excluded as a possibility (e.g., because of very low PID-5-VRIN scale scores) but PID-5-ORS scores suggest that the respondent may have overreported personality pathology, PID-5 trait and domain profiles should be interpreted with caution. PID-5-ORS scores of 3 or greater do not necessarily imply that the test taker is free of psychopathology; indeed, personality psychopathology and overreporting are not mutually exclusive. As mentioned previously, overreporting could occur for different reasons, and these reasons should be investigated depending on the context of the evaluation, collecting collateral and other additional information. For instance, high scores on the PID-5-ORS could be associated with actual severe personality psychopathology, a need to be taken seriously, or the person's desire to appear as though they have a severe mental disorder. From this perspective, researchers may or may not choose to exclude participants scoring high on the PID-5-ORS, whereas clinicians may want to collect data regarding the history or current corroborating evidence of personality dysfunction or psychopathology.

Table 4–2. Personality Inventory for DSM-5 Over-Reporting Scale (PID-5-ORS) items

PID-5 scales	PID-5-ORS items
Hostility	170
Restricted affectivity	8
Depressivity	178
Suspiciousness	2
Callousness	166
Grandiosity	40
Risk taking	39
Irresponsibility	171
Cognitive and perceptual dysregulation	44
Unusual beliefs and experiences	150

Note. PID-5 item numbers refer to the 220-item version of the instrument.

In summary, the PID-5-ORS seems to provide a clinically useful tool for recognizing respondents who tend to exaggerate the description of their personality pathology. The PID-5-ORS cannot provide any information about the reasons leading a test taker to provide a potentially exaggerated description of their dysfunctional personality traits; additional clinical or forensic work would be necessary to clarify the motivations and implications for PID-5-ORS score elevation.

Positive Impression Management and Underreported Psychopathology

Positive Impression Management

Just as with negative impression management, the tendency to minimize psychopathology or dissimulate optimal psychological functioning can also threaten the interpretation of self-report measures (e.g., Rogers and Bender 2018). Failure to recognize underreporting of psychopathology can result in biased interpretations of test responses, potentially leading to inaccurate clinical assessment and misdiagnosis (e.g., Sellbom and Bagby 2008). Underreporting or positive impression management refers to an unexpectedly low level of endorsement of items indicating psychopathology or an unexpectedly high level of endorsements of items indicating adaptive functioning given an individual's actual level of psychopathology (e.g., Butcher et al. 2001).

Available data suggest that psychological measures are generally susceptible to positive impression management in numerous settings (for a review, see Rogers and Bender 2018); not surprisingly, the PID-5 is not an exception (Dhillon et al. 2017; McGee Ng et al. 2016). Blanchard and Farber (2016) carried out a study on 547 former or current therapy patients and found that 54% of the patients minimized how badly they really felt and 39% underreported the severity of their symptoms. Positive impression management or underreporting may stem from a variety of processes and causes, such as avoidance of difficulties; identity concerns; competitiveness; or attainment of external rewards, such as when convincing a court that dysfunctional personality characteristics are not at issue when parents are undergoing child custody evaluations (e.g., Rogers and Bender 2018).

Although the denial of negative characteristics and the presentation of positive characteristics are both forms of socially desirable responding, they reflect distinct, dissociable processes that can be interpreted differently in applied settings (Rogers and Bender 2018; Williams et al. 2019). A defensive or avoidant attitude characterizes individuals denying psychological symptoms and impairment, tending to minimize psychological difficulties (Rogers and Bender 2018). By contrast, other individuals misrepresent themselves by providing an extremely positive impression, putting forth an exaggeratedly positive image through endorsement of positive attributes; this response style can be diffuse and is not limited to denial of psychopathology per se (Rogers and Bender 2018).

PID-5 Positive Impression Management Response Distortion Scale

Against this background, Williams and colleagues (2019) developed the PID-5 Positive Impression Management Response Distortion (PID-5-PRD) scale, which aimed to distinguish between underreporters and genuine responders on the PID-5. Williams et al. (2019) recruited a sample of 106 psychiatric inpatients and asked them to complete the PID-5 twice. The first time, the PID-5 was administered under standard instructions (i.e., genuine responses), whereas in the second administration, participants were assigned to one of two conditions in which they were required to either deny pathological personality traits or present with adaptive personality traits.

In order to develop the PID-5-PRD scale, Williams et al. (2019) examined item combinations and focused on item pairs that were moderately correlated among simulators but were virtually uncorrelated for genuine respondents. The rationale for this selection strategy was to identify patterns of correlation between items induced by underreporting and positive impression management.

As a result of this procedure, 11 pairs of nonredundant PID-5 items were selected to be included in the PID-5-PRD. These 11 items are listed in Table 4–3. The PID-5-PRD total score is obtained by summing the responses to these 22 PID-5 items; thus, the PID-5-PRD score ranges from 0 to 66. Williams et al. (2019) proposed that PID-5-PRD scores greater than 20 are suggestive of likely genuine responding; PID-5-PRD scores less than 11 are suggestive of underreporting or positive impression management; and PID-5-PRD scores ranging from 11 to 20 cannot be clearly inferred to reflect either underreporting or genuine responding.

In the U.S. normative sample, scores on the PID-5-PRD ranged from 0 to 55, with a mean score of 11.50 and an SD of 7.88. PID-5-PRD scores were correlated 0.37 with PID-5-VRIN scale scores and 0.43 with PID-5-ORS scores. Approximately 61% of participants in the normative sample scored lower than the suggested cutoff of 11, and 12.5% scored above the cutoff of 20.

Table 4–3. Personality Inventory for DSM-5 Positive Impression Management Response Distortion (PID-5-PRD) scale items

PID-5 scales	PID-5-PRD items[a]
Anxiousness	96[b]
Emotional lability	122
Hostility	38
Depressivity	119, 148, 163, 168, 169
Suspiciousness	2
Withdrawal	136
Callousness	11, 183, 198
Manipulativeness	162
Distractibility	47, 199
Risk taking	98[b]
Cognitive and perceptual dysregulation	36, 42, 154, 192
Unusual beliefs and experiences	106

[a]PID-5 item numbers refer to the 220-item version of the instrument.
[b]Reverse-scored item.

The results of Williams et al.'s (2019) study support the potential usefulness of the PID-5-PRD in screening for positive impression management, but additional study is needed to understand the scale's properties in different scenarios. A very large proportion of individuals in the normative sample obtained scores below the cutoff suggested for identification of positive impression management, and an even larger proportion scored within the low to indeterminate range. Use of these cutoffs in settings other than those similar to Williams et al.'s (2019) study (i.e., psychiatric inpatients) may result in many individuals being misidentified as engaging in positive impression management. As is the case with overreporting, differentiating intentional from unintentional underreporting requires collecting collateral data and additional information. PID-5-PRD scores should never be used as confirmation of positive impression management responding. When present, positive impression management may result from a variety of factors, such as having extremely conservative attitudes or simply being extremely well adjusted.

Williams et al. (2019) further attempted to construct an index differentiating between the two forms of positive impression management: denial of negative characteristics (which they referred to as *defensive responding*) and exaggeration of positive characteristics (which they referred to as *social desirability responding*). The authors focused on rates of total denial responses (i.e., endorsement of "very false" responses on PID-5 items) in their two positive impression management conditions, identifying items for which "very false" was endorsed much more frequently in the exaggerated positive characteristic condition than in the denial condition. The authors identified 17 such items, listed in Table 4–4. Summing the responses keyed in the direction of endorsement rather than denial (i.e., "very false," "often false," "often true," or "very true," keyed as 0, 1, 2, and 3, respectively) produces an index ranging from 0 to 51 that can be used to distinguish between exaggerated positive presentation and denial of psychopathology. Williams et al. (2019) proposed that scores on the index less than 12 are suggestive of exaggerated positive presentation, and scores greater than 18 are indicative of defensiveness.

Some caution is required in interpreting the items in this index, however. First, the items in this index all generally refer to psychopathology, so in an important sense the index reflects different forms of denial behavior (or, equivalently, endorsement behavior) rather than denial of negative content versus endorsement of positive content per se. Second, some items on the index are not in the PID-5-PRD, raising questions about how to best interpret the index vis-à-vis that scale.

Table 4–4. Personality Inventory for DSM-5 (PID-5) items differing in endorsement rates between types of positive impression management conditions

PID-5 scales	Items[a]
Anxiousness	93
Emotional lability	18
Hostility	38
Perseveration	80
Separation insecurity	50, 57
Anhedonia	23, 30[b]
Withdrawal	82
Depressivity	66
Suspiciousness	2
Impulsivity	4
Distractibility	68, 88
Eccentricity	52
Cognitive and perceptual dysregulation	193
Unusual beliefs and experiences	209

[a]PID-5 item numbers refer to the 220-item version of the instrument.
[b]Reverse-scored item.

EFFECTS OF IMPRESSION MANAGEMENT ON PID-5 TRAIT AND DOMAIN SCALES

As described earlier, several studies have attempted to model the effect of response bias and impression management on PID-5 trait and domain scales. Although these studies have used different methodologies (e.g., experimentally induced response bias vs. observationally identified response bias), certain patterns have emerged whereby some scales appear to be more affected by typical response bias patterns than others. These patterns may be useful to clinicians and other users of the PID-5 in identifying and characterizing response bias and impression management in respondents.

Table 4–5 presents descriptive statistics showing differences in PID-5 trait and domain scale scores between genuine or credibly responding groups and response bias groups across six samples from four studies

Table 4–5. Standardized differences in PID-5 trait and domain scales in response bias groups relative to credibly responding groups

	NIM		PIM	
	Mean *d*	SD *d*	Mean *d*	SD *d*
Trait scales				
Anhedonia	1.26	0.23	−1.03	0.83
Anxiousness	1.01	0.39	−1.30	0.81
Attention seeking	0.23	0.14	−0.28	0.44
Callousness	1.06	0.55	−0.42	0.19
Deceitfulness	0.88	0.33	−0.75	0.21
Depressivity	1.51	0.41	−1.12	0.83
Distractibility	0.96	0.17	−1.31	0.94
Eccentricity	1.15	0.50	−0.94	0.65
Emotional lability	0.94	0.22	−1.20	0.84
Grandiosity	0.43	0.37	−0.01	0.40
Hostility	0.99	0.36	−1.10	0.52
Impulsivity	0.81	0.31	−1.10	0.75
Intimacy avoidance	0.78	0.43	−0.18	0.28
Irresponsibility	1.25	0.50	−0.90	0.55
Manipulativeness	0.52	0.32	−0.47	0.12
Cognitive and perceptual dysregulation	1.47	0.55	−0.80	0.60
Perseveration	1.10	0.25	−1.01	0.65
Restricted affectivity	0.10	0.59	−0.29	0.16
Rigid perfectionism	−0.25	0.48	0.09	0.25
Risk taking	0.18	0.30	−0.48	0.36
Separation insecurity	0.62	0.32	−0.74	0.30
Submissiveness	0.22	0.20	−0.30	0.16
Suspiciousness	1.50	0.49	−0.90	0.84
Unusual beliefs and experiences	1.10	0.57	−0.55	0.34
Withdrawal	1.07	0.41	−0.87	0.74
Mean absolute value	0.85	0.38	0.73	0.51

Table 4–5. Standardized differences in PID-5 trait and domain scales in response bias groups relative to credibly responding groups *(continued)*

	NIM		PIM	
	Mean *d*	SD *d*	Mean *d*	SD *d*
Domain scales				
Negative affectivity	1.23	0.28	–1.35	0.71
Detachment	1.33	0.43	–0.85	0.68
Antagonism	0.78	0.47	–0.54	0.17
Disinhibition	1.20	0.09	–1.38	0.80
Psychoticism	1.37	0.58	–0.90	0.62
Mean absolute value	1.08	0.27	1.00	0.60

Note. NIM=negative impression management; PID-5=Personality Inventory for DSM-5; PIM=positive impression management.

(McGee Ng et al. 2016; Quilty et al. 2018; Sellbom et al. 2018; Williams et al. 2019). Two of the studies examined response bias effects by using preexisting validity scales to identify groups of individuals likely to be overreporting, underreporting, or credibly reporting (McGee Ng et al. 2016; Quilty et al. 2018); two other studies induced response biases experimentally by means of instructed responding (Sellbom et al. 2018; Williams et al. 2019). The values in Table 4–5 are average mean differences between groups across studies, expressed in *d* statistics (i.e., SDs), where a positive value means that the impression management group had higher scores compared with the credibly responding group and a negative value means that the impression management group had lower scores compared with the credibly responding group.

As can be seen in Table 4–5, the trait and domain scales varied substantially in their change with impression management. The changes in overreporting and underreporting are highly correlated across scales ($r=–0.72$), suggesting that scores that tend to increase with overreporting will also decrease with underreporting.

Scores on the Attention Seeking, Grandiosity, Restricted Affectivity, Rigid Perfectionism, and Submissiveness scales seem to change less with impression management overall than do scores on the other scales. Risk Taking scores change less with negative impression management, and Intimacy Avoidance scores change less with positive impression management. Rigid Perfectionism is noteworthy in that under impression management it tends to change slightly in the opposite direction from the other trait scales. As Williams et al. (2019) noted, individuals approaching the PID-5 from an impression management perspective may interpret the item content of these seven scales somewhat differently than individuals approaching the items candidly; another possibility is that from a social desirability perspective the content of these scales is more neutral than that of other scales.

Among the domain scales, Negative Affectivity had the largest changes with impression management and Antagonism the smallest changes. The smaller changes of Antagonism with impression management might be surprising, although this domain does include scales such as Grandiosity, which was the least susceptible to impression management of all the trait scales.

RESPONSE VALIDITY, INFORMANTS, AND THE PERSONALITY INVENTORY FOR DSM-5— INFORMANT FORM

Collateral information is critical when evaluating possible invalidity in responses, whether the concerns are about inconsistent responding or systematic response bias. Although this collateral information can take many forms, such as from records or behavioral observation, key information often is obtained from informants such as friends, family, partners, health care staff, or other individuals with knowledge of the respondent. The PID-5—Informant Form (PID-5-IRF) quantifies informant perceptions of the respondent, and therefore it can be useful in characterizing possible sources of invalidity in self-reported PID-5 responses.

Quilty et al. (2018) examined differences in PID-5-IRF scores and differences in correspondence between the self-report form of the PID-5 (PID-5-SRF) and the PID-5-IRF among groups of individuals identified on the basis of external response validity scales as likely underreporting, overreporting, or credibly reporting on the PID-5-SRF. In general, Quilty et al. (2018) found that PID-5-IRF scores appeared to vary less with response bias than did PID-5-SRF scores, especially in the case of underreporting. There was a tendency for informants' responses to track patterns of validity scales—individuals identified as overreporting were likely to be rated by informants as having more psychopathology, and individuals identified as underreporting were likely to be rated by informants as having less psychopathology—but the differences across response bias groups on the informant form were relatively modest compared with responses on the self-report form. Agreement between informants and respondents did not vary with degree of inferred response bias, except for the Psychoticism domain score, which was characterized by higher levels of agreement among cases of underreporting respondents.

Overall, Quilty et al.'s (2018) results suggest that the PID-5-IRF can be a useful additional source of information in assessing respondents when response invalidity is a concern. Their results underscored that in many cases, putative overreporting or underreporting as reflected in self-report validity scales may actually reflect genuinely high or low levels of psychopathology and not necessarily response distortion per se. Their results also suggest that the PID-5-IRF may be especially useful when there are concerns about underreporting on the PID-5-SRF.

Of course, informant responses are susceptible to possible inconsistency and response biases as well. For example, individuals may be volunteering to complete the PID-5-IRF on behalf of an acquaintance, friend, or loved one and may not attend as closely as they would on a self-report form affecting their own outcomes. Also, if an informant has an ongoing relationship with the respondent and their responses could be reasonably inferred in a clinical report or feedback session, they may be motivated to respond differently than if their responses were kept confidential or obscured. Finally, each informant has a unique perspective on the respondent for various reasons, and this should be considered when interpreting informant reports.

CONCLUSION

The development of the embedded validity scales to assess different response styles for the PID-5 trait and domain scale scores has allowed clinicians and researchers to screen for possible invalidity in responses. Validity scales have the potential to improve the utility of the PID-5 in applied professional settings, particularly in those settings where reasons for distorted responses or response biases might be salient (e.g., forensic evaluations; Hopwood and Sellbom 2013). Of course, a comprehensive clinical assessment of response styles is always recommended and needed; no validity scale alone can provide assessors with certainty that a response distortion process is in place. The accuracy of validity scales depends on the base rates and prevalence of inconsistent and biased responses in a given setting (e.g., Sellbom et al. 2018; Somma et al. 2018), which require knowledge of the clinical context in which the assessment occurs. Collateral information and additional data should always be collected, and PID-5 validity scale scores should be considered in the context of a comprehensive psychological assessment. In addition to the validity scales, users should consider the PID-5-IRF as an additional source of information about self-presentation on the PID-5. The PID-5 represents a relatively new and constantly evolving instrument; accordingly, cross-validation and extension of the research data on the PID-5 validity scales are essential.

REFERENCES

Al-Dajani N, Gralnick TM, Bagby RM: A psychometric review of the Personality Inventory for DSM-5 (PID-5): current status and future directions. J Pers Assess 98(1):62–81, 2016 26619968

American Psychiatric Association: Diagnostic and Statistical Manual of Mental Disorders, 5th Edition. Washington, DC, American Psychiatric Association, 2013

Bagby RM, Psych C, Quilty LC, et al: Personality and depression. Can J Psychiatry 53(1):14–25, 2008 18286868

Blanchard M, Farber BA: Lying in psychotherapy: why and what clients don't tell their therapist about therapy and their relationship. Couns Psychol Q 29:90–112, 2016

Bowling NA, Huang JL, Bragg CB, et al: Who cares and who is careless? Insufficient effort responding as a reflection of respondent personality. J Pers Soc Psychol 111(2):218–229, 2016 26927958

Burchett D, Bagby RM: Multimethod assessment of distortion: integrating data from interviews, collateral records, and standardized assessment tools, in Multimethod Clinical Assessment. Edited by Hopwood CJ, Bornstein RF. New York, Guilford, 2014, pp 345–378

Burchett DL, Ben-Porath YS: The impact of overreporting on MMPI-2-RF substantive scale score validity. Assessment 17(4):497–516, 2010 20739584

Butcher JN, Graham JR, Ben-Porath YS, et al: MMPI-2: Minnesota Multiphasic Personality Inventory-2: Manual for Administration and Scoring, Revised Edition. Minneapolis, University of Minnesota Press, 2001

Curran PG: Methods for the detection of carelessly invalid responses in survey data. J Exp Soc Psychol 66:4–19, 2016

Dhillon S, Bagby RM, Kushner SC, et al: The impact of underreporting and overreporting on the validity of the Personality Inventory for DSM-5 (PID-5): a simulation analog design investigation. Psychol Assess 29(4):473–478, 2017 27414150

Hopwood CJ, Sellbom M: Implications of DSM-5 personality traits for forensic psychology. Psychol Inj Law 6:314–323, 2013

Keeley JW, Webb C, Peterson D, et al: Development of a response inconsistency scale for the Personality Inventory for DSM-5. J Pers Assess 98(4):351–359, 2016 27049169

Lowmaster SE, Hartman MJ, Zimmermann J, et al: Further validation of the response inconsistency scale for the Personality Inventory for DSM-5. J Pers Assess 102(6):743–750, 2020 31625765

Lowmaster SE, Hartman MJ, Zimmermann J, et al: Further validation of the response inconsistency scale for the Personality Inventory for DSM-5 (correction). J Pers Assess 103(4):571, 2021 33970722

Maniaci MR, Rogge RD: Caring about carelessness: participant inattention and its effects on research. J Res Pers 48:61–83, 2014

Maples JL, Carter NT, Few LR, et al: Testing whether the DSM-5 personality disorder trait model can be measured with a reduced set of items: an item response theory investigation of the Personality Inventory for DSM-5. Psychol Assess 27(4):1195–1210, 2015 25844534

McGee Ng SA, Bagby RM, Goodwin BE, et al: The effect of response bias on the Personality Inventory for DSM-5 (PID-5). J Pers Assess 98(1):51–61, 2016 26583767

Meade AW, Craig SB: Identifying careless responses in survey data. Psychol Methods 17(3):437–455, 2012 22506584

Quilty LC, Cosentino N, Bagby RM: Response bias and the Personality Inventory for DSM-5: contrasting self- and informant-report. Pers Disord 9(4):346–353, 2018 28368145

Rogers R, Bender SD: Clinical Assessment of Malingering and Deception, 4th Edition. New York, Guilford, 2018

Sellbom M, Bagby RM: Response styles on multiscale inventories, in Clinical Assessment of Malingering and Deception. Edited by Rogers R. New York, Guilford, 2008, pp 182–206

Sellbom M, Dhillon S, Bagby RM: Development and validation of an Overreporting Scale for the Personality Inventory for DSM-5 (PID-5). Psychol Assess 30(5):582–593, 2018 28557479

Somma A, Borroni S, Kelley SE, et al: Further evidence for the validity of a response inconsistency scale for the Personality Inventory for DSM-5 in Italian community-dwelling adolescents, community-dwelling adults, and clinical adults. Psychol Assess 30(7):929–940, 2018 29565615

Williams MM, Rogers R, Sharf AJ, et al: Faking good: an investigation of social desirability and defensiveness in an inpatient sample with personality disorder traits. J Pers Assess 101(3):253–263, 2019 29717901

CHAPTER 5

Special Applications of the PID-5

The Personality Inventory for DSM-5 (PID-5; American Psychiatric Association 2013) is an evolving assessment instrument; new scales and scoring methods are constantly being developed either to facilitate translation and communication between different diagnostic systems (e.g., the *International Classification of Diseases*, 11th Revision [ICD-11]) or to assess specific personality variables (e.g., psychopathy). In this chapter, different versions of and scoring methods for the PID-5 are presented in order to allow clinicians and researchers to select the optimal version and scoring method of the PID-5 for specific application and assessment needs.

HARMONIZING TWO DIAGNOSTIC SYSTEMS: ASSESSING ICD-11 PERSONALITY DOMAINS USING THE PID-5

ICD-11 embraced a complete redefinition of the diagnosis of personality disorders, including a fully dimensional classification system for personality disorders. The ICD-11 and DSM-5 Alternative Model for Personality Disorders (AMPD) approaches to personality disorder diagnosis are comparable overall with respect to both severity and trait descriptors except for the trait domain of psychoticism. Specifically, the ICD-11 model focuses on general personality disorder diagnostic requirements (i.e., primary diagnosis), followed by assessment of the severity of personality pathology (i.e., personality difficulty, mild personality disorder, moderate personality disorder, severe personality disorder) and then offers the opportunity to describe the degree to which each individual expresses characteristics listed in the five trait domains (i.e., trait domain specifiers).

ICD-11 trait domains describe the most prominent aspects of the subject's personality that contribute to personality dysfunction (World Health Organization 2023). The ICD-11 and AMPD domains are conceptually aligned with one another (e.g., Bach and Mulder 2022a, 2022b; Mulder et al. 2011; Widiger and Simonsen 2005), and available data (e.g., Bach et al. 2018; Crego and Widiger 2020; Oltmanns and Widiger 2018; Somma et al. 2020) have shown that the AMPD and ICD-11 trait domains converge and capture the same constructs. Indeed, the ICD-11 five trait domains show theoretically and conceptually expected associations with the DSM-5 AMPD domains (e.g., Bach and Mulder 2022a, 2022b; McCabe and Widiger 2020). Table 5–1 lists ICD-11 domains and provides a short description of each domain.

As is apparent in Table 5–1, four of the five domains of ICD-11 are closely aligned with four of the five domains of DSM-5 Section III (Mulder et al. 2016). Specifically, the ICD-11 negative affectivity, detachment, dissociality, and disinhibition domains are isomorphic with the DSM-5 AMPD negative affectivity, detachment, antagonism, and disinhibition domains, respectively. However, the ICD-11 dimensional trait model does not include a domain meant to describe the cognitive and perceptual features of schizotypy (i.e., psychoticism in DSM-5 AMPD), but it includes an anankastia dimension not included in the final DSM-5 AMPD (American Psychiatric Association 2013).

The absence of psychoticism in the ICD-11 model of personality disorder is consistent with the placement of schizotypal personality disorder under the "Schizophrenia or Other Primary Psychotic Disorders" section in ICD-11. Moreover, it should be observed that although the final DSM-5 AMPD model does not include the anankastia domain, compulsivity is represented by the pathological trait of rigid perfectionism (e.g., Bach and Mulder 2022b; Bach and Zine El Abiddine 2020; Watters and Bagby 2018). Additionally, it is worth noting that although the inclusion of traits within each ICD-11 domain was considered, the ICD-11 Working Group believed that their inclusion would result in unnecessary and undesirable complexity in the proposal (Mulder et al. 2011; Tyrer 2012; Tyrer et al. 2011). Thus, a notable difference between the

Table 5–1. Description and typical manifestations of ICD-11 trait domains

ICD-11 trait domain	Description	Examples of manifestations
Negative affectivity	Tendency to experience a wide range of negative emotions	Experiencing a wide range of negative emotions of an intensity and frequency disproportionate to the situation that generated them Emotional lability and poor emotional regulation A negativistic attitude Low self-esteem and self-confidence Suspiciousness
Detachment	Tendency to maintain interpersonal distance (social detachment) and emotional distance (emotional detachment)	Social detachment (avoidance of social interactions, absence of friendships, and avoidance of intimacy) Emotional detachment (discretion, detachment, and limited emotional expression and experience)
Dissociality	Absence of consideration for others' rights and feelings, including both self-centeredness and lack of empathy	Egocentric perspective (e.g., attitude of pretension; expectation of admiration; attention-seeking behaviors; exclusive concern for one's own needs, desires, and well-being and not that of others) Lack of empathy (e.g., indifference to the fact that one's actions may hurt others, deceitfulness, manipulative behavior, exploitation of others, malice and physical aggression, callousness regarding others' suffering, unscrupulousness in order to achieve one's goals)

Table 5–1. Description and typical manifestations of ICD-11 trait domains *(continued)*

ICD-11 trait domain	Description	Examples of manifestations
Disinhibition	Tendency to act thoughtlessly on the basis of external or internal (i.e., feelings, emotions, thoughts) stimuli without considering the potential negative consequences	Impulsivity Irresponsible distractibility Thoughtlessness Lack of planning
Anankastia	Exclusive focus on one's own standards of perfection with respect to right and wrong and control over one's own and others' behavior and situations to ensure compliance with these standards	Perfectionism (e.g., preoccupation with social rules and duties; scrupulous attention to detail, routines, excessive planning and organization, order and cleanliness) Emotional and behavioral self-control (e.g., rigid control over emotional expression, stubbornness, inflexibility, perseveration)

diagnostic model of personality disorders in ICD-11 and that in the DSM-5 AMPD is that the five ICD-11 domains do not include any trait scales (Tyrer et al. 2015). The rationale for this choice is related to the policies of the World Health Organization, which emphasized that the ICD-11 personality disorder classification system also should be viable and useful for health care professionals working in resource-limited facilities (International Advisory Group for the Revision of ICD-10 Mental and Behavioural Disorders 2011).

Assessing ICD-11 Domains Through PID-5 Trait Scales

As soon as the first operationalization of the now official ICD-11 trait domain specifiers was available, Bach and colleagues (2017) developed an algorithm for computing ICD-11 trait domain scores on the basis of the administration of the PID-5. The proposal of Bach et al. (2017) aimed at facilitating the dialogue between the two diagnostic systems (i.e., DSM-5 and ICD-11) and could be particularly useful for PID-5 users who need to adapt their personality assessment to ICD-11 personality disorder diagnoses.

Different studies have shown the usefulness of this algorithm (for a review, see Bach and Mulder 2022b) and supported its use as a clinical tool for assessing dysfunctional personality trait domains according to the ICD-11 model of personality disorders. The algorithm for computing the ICD-11 domain scales using the PID-5 trait scales is detailed in Table 5–2.

Table 5–2. Algorithms for computing the ICD-11 domain scales using the Personality Inventory for DSM-5 (PID-5) trait scales

A. ICD-11 domains	B. PID-5 trait scales	C. Sum of trait scores	D. Overall average score (total of column C divided by the number of traits listed in column B)
Negative affectivity	Emotional lability		
	Anxiousness		
	Depressivity		
Detachment	Withdrawal		
	Intimacy avoidance		
	Restricted affectivity		
Dissociality	Callousness		
	Grandiosity		
	Manipulativeness		
	Hostility		
Disinhibition	Irresponsibility		
	Impulsivity		
	Distractibility		
	Risk taking		
Anankastia	Rigid perfectionism		
	Perseveration		

Note. Traits given in column B identify the trait scales of the 220-item version of the PID-5.

As is illustrated in Table 5–2, 16 PID-5 traits (i.e., 158 PID-5 items) were designated to generate the 5 ICD-11 domain scores (Bach et al. 2017). This approach to the assessment of ICD-11 domains was found to be useful both in the United States (e.g., Sellbom et al. 2020) and across the world (e.g., Fang et al. 2021; Hemmati et al. 2021; Lotfi et al. 2018; Lugo et al. 2019), supporting the usefulness of the PID-5 for new purposes beyond its original intention.

Versions of the PID-5 Specifically Developed to Assess ICD-11 Domains

Because resources are often limited in both clinical and research contexts, lengthy measures for maladaptive personality trait domains (e.g., 158 items for computing the PID-5/ICD-11 domain scores) may be more time-consuming than desired. In order to overcome these difficulties and promote the widespread adoption of dimensional models of dysfunctional domains assessment, Kerber et al. (2022) developed a 34-item version of the PID-5 called the Personality Inventory for DSM-5— Brief Form Plus (PID-5-BF+). This brief measure is aimed at efficiently assessing the dysfunctional personality domains of both DSM-5 and ICD-11 personality disorder models. Indeed, this version of the PID-5 was explicitly developed to facilitate the translation between ICD-11 and DSM-5 models of personality disorders.

Kerber et al. (2022) recruited large samples of English- and German-speaking participants ($N=2,927$) and used data from these individuals to develop a measure of the ICD-11 and DSM-5 dysfunctional personality domains, including the DSM-5 psychoticism domain. Kerber et al. (2022) relied on the item pool of the 220-item version of the PID-5 and applied ant colony optimization algorithms to generate a maximally valid and reliable measure of the ICD-11/DSM-5 AMPD domains.

Table 5–3 lists the PID-5 items included in the PID-5-BF+, and the scoring algorithm for computing ICD-11/DSM-5 domains relying on the PID-5-BF+ trait scales is provided in Table 5–4.

The resulting self-report measure (i.e., the PID-5-BF+) was composed of 34 items measuring 6 maladaptive trait domains (i.e., negative affectivity, detachment, dissociality, disinhibition, anankastia, and psychoticism) and 17 traits. As in the PID-5, each PID-5-BF+ item is rated on a 4-point scale, ranging from "0=very false or often false" to "3=very true or often true."

Notably, Kerber et al.'s (2022) study showed that the PID-5-BF+ demonstrated adequate internal consistency reliability and factor struc-

Table 5–3. Personality Inventory for DSM-5 (PID-5) items included in the PID-5—Brief Form Plus (PID-5-BF+)

A. DSM-5/ICD-11 traits computed with the PID-5-BF+	B. PID-5 item number	C. Mean of item scores
Anxiousness	109, 110	
Emotional lability	62, 122	
Separation insecurity	50, 64	
Withdrawal	82, 136	
Anhedonia	23, 189	
Intimacy avoidance	89, 108	
Manipulativeness	162, 219	
Deceitfulness	126, 218	
Grandiosity	187, 197	
Irresponsibility	129, 160	
Impulsivity	4, 17	
Distractibility	6, 132	
Rigid perfectionism	123, 176	
Perseveration	60, 128	
Unusual beliefs and experiences	194, 209	
Eccentricity	25, 185	
Perceptual dysregulation	44, 77	

Note. PID-5 item numbers in column B refer to the 220-item version of the PID-5.

ture and strong convergent and adequate discriminant validity. Additionally, the criterion validity of the PID-5-BF+ was supported by meaningful correlations between PID-5-BF+ domain scores and Big Five personality traits and between ICD-11 maladaptive trait domains and interpersonal distress (Kerber et al. 2022). Additionally, in Kerber et al.'s (2022) study, the PID-5-BF+ negative affectivity and disinhibition domain scores were able to differentiate between clinical participants with and without a borderline personality disorder diagnosis. Finally, PID-5-BF+ negative affectivity, detachment, and psychoticism domain scale scores significantly differentiated between mild and more severe mental health internalizing conditions without a personality disorder diagnosis (Kerber et al. 2022).

Table 5–4.   Personality Inventory for DSM-5—Brief Form Plus (PID-5-BF+), trait domain scale scoring

A. DSM-5/ICD-11 domains	B. PID-5-BF+ trait scales	C. Sum of trait scores	D. Overall average score (total of column C divided by the number of traits listed in column B)
Negative affectivity	Anxiousness		
	Emotional lability		
	Separation insecurity		
Detachment	Anhedonia		
	Withdrawal		
	Intimacy avoidance		
Dissociality	Grandiosity		
	Manipulativeness		
	Deceitfulness		
Disinhibition	Impulsivity		
	Irresponsibility		
	Distractibility		
Anankastia	Rigid perfectionism		
	Perseveration		
Psychoticism	Unusual beliefs and experiences		
	Eccentricity		
	Perceptual dysregulation		

The development of brief but reliable and valid measures to assess pathological personality domains according to different models (i.e., DSM-5 AMPD and ICD-11) is critical for adopting dimensional models of personality pathology in both clinical and research contexts. In line with these considerations, Bach et al. (2020) promoted a transcultural validation project of a modified version of the PID-5-BF+, the 36-item PID-5-BF+ Modified (PID-5-BF+M). The PID-5-BF+M operationalizes the DSM-5 and ICD-11 domains using three primary traits per domain so that all domains are represented by a comparable number of indicators. The main difference from the version developed by Kerber et al. (2022) is related to the definition of the anankastia domain. Specifically, Bach et al. (2020) proposed assessing anankastia using the items originally designed to assess the traits of perfectionism, rigidity, and order (Krueger et al. 2012), which were later merged into the rigid perfectionism domain in favor of parsimony on the basis of the results of factor analyses (Krueger et al. 2012).

Table 5–5 lists the PID-5 items included in the PID-5-BF+M. Table 5–6 presents the scoring for computing the ICD-11 dysfunctional personality domains according to the PID-5-BF+M.

Table 5–5. Personality Inventory for DSM-5 (PID-5) items included in the PID-5—Brief Form Plus Modified (PID-5-BF+M)

A. ICD-11 traits computed with the PID-5-BF+ of Bach et al. (2020)	B. PID-5 item	C. Mean of item scores
Anxiousness	109, 110	
Emotional lability	62, 122	
Separation insecurity	50, 64	
Withdrawal	82, 136	
Anhedonia	23, 189	
Intimacy avoidance	89, 108	
Manipulativeness	162, 219	
Deceitfulness	126, 218	
Grandiosity	187, 197	
Irresponsibility	129, 160	
Impulsiveness	4, 17	
Distractibility	6, 132	
Perfectionism	123, 176	
Rigidity	140, 220	
Orderliness	34, 115	
Unusual beliefs and experiences	194, 209	
Eccentricity	25, 185	
Perceptual dysregulation	44, 77	

Note. PID-5 item numbers in column B refer to the 220-item version of the PID-5.

Table 5–6. Personality Inventory for DSM-5 and ICD-11 Plus Modified (PID-5-BF+M) trait domain scale scoring

A. ICD-11 domains	B. PID-5-BF+ trait scales	C. Sum of trait scores	D. Overall average score (total of column C divided by the number of traits listed in column B)
Negative affectivity	Anxiousness		
	Emotional lability		
	Separation insecurity		
Detachment	Anhedonia		
	Withdrawal		
	Intimacy avoidance		
Dissociality	Grandiosity		
	Manipulativeness		
	Deceitfulness		
Disinhibition	Impulsivity		
	Irresponsibility		
	Distractibility		
Anankastia	Perfectionism		
	Rigidity		
	Orderliness		
Psychoticism	Unusual beliefs and experiences		
	Eccentricity		
	Perceptual dysregulation		

The PID-5-BF+M showed adequate psychometric properties and transcultural validity across 17 samples and 12 languages (Bach et al. 2020). This measure is particularly useful when clinicians and researchers need to focus on the ICD-11 approach to the diagnosis of personality disorders and when they are interested in assessing anankastia/compulsivity in greater detail, such as when obsessive-compulsive features are prominent (e.g., Crego et al. 2015). The DSM-5 AMPD trait system describes features of anankastia in terms of low levels of disinhibition (i.e., high scores on rigid perfectionism and perseveration).

ADAPTATIONS OF THE PID-5 FOR THE ASSESSMENT OF FORENSIC CONSTRUCTS

From the initial publication of the PID-5, different adaptations for forensic contexts have been developed by various research groups on the basis of specific assessment needs. The PID-5 Triarchic (PID-5-Tri) scales and PID-5 Forensic Faceted Brief Form (PID-5-FFBF) are examples.

PID-5 Triarchic Scales

In order to provide a sound measure for the assessment of psychopathy, Drislane et al. (2019) focused on the PID-5 item pool to develop scales designed to assess dimensions of the triarchic model of psychopathy (Patrick et al. 2009) on the basis of the AMPD trait model. The triarchic model of psychopathy was proposed by Patrick et al. (2009) as a psychopathological and developmental model of psychopathy, comprising constructs deduced from the available literature on psychopathy and represented to varying degrees across different conceptualizations of psychopathy (e.g., Patrick and Drislane 2015). The triarchic model of psychopathy includes three main dimensions: 1) boldness, defined as the intersection of high dominance, low anxiety, and recklessness; 2) meanness, reflecting tendencies toward callousness, cruelty, predatory aggression, and excitement-seeking; and 3) disinhibition, assessing impulsivity, irresponsibility, oppositionality, and anger and hostility.

The computational algorithm for computing the PID-5-Boldness, PID-5-Meanness, and PID-5-Disinhibition scales using the 220-item version of PID-5 is shown in Table 5–7.

The PID-5-Tri scales can be computed easily after the administration of the 220-item version of the PID-5 whenever clinicians and researchers find it useful to describe their patients' personality in terms of the triarchic model of psychopathy. The PID-5-Tri scale items were selected from the PID-5 item pool on the basis of a construct rating and scale refinement approach (for a detailed description, see Drislane et al. 2019). Specifically, Drislane et al.'s (2019) study included a sample ($N=210$) from which the scales were developed and an independent community validation sample ($N=240$) recruited to have elevated psychopathic traits. The PID-5-Tri scales showed adequate reliability and construct validity, as evidenced by meaningful associations with other measures

Table 5–7. Personality Inventory for DSM-5 (PID-5) items included in the PID-5 Triarchic scales

A. PID-5 Triarchic scales	B. PID-5 item	C. Sum of the scores of the items listed in column B	D. Average score (total from column C divided by the total number of items listed in column B)
PID-5-Boldness (15 items)	7(R), 15(R), 65, 87(R), 95(R), 96, 107, 111, 130(R), 155, 180, 186(R), 195, 202(R), 211		
PID-5-Meanness (21 items)	8, 10, 13, 40, 54, 72, 73, 84, 90(R), 91, 97(R), 102(R), 116, 153, 166, 167, 183, 184, 200, 207, 208		
PID-5-Disinhibition (19 items)	3, 4, 16, 17, 28, 31, 58(R), 103, 126, 129, 134, 156, 158, 160, 171, 190, 201, 204, 210(R)		

Note. PID-5 item numbers in column B refer to the 220-item version of the PID-5; (R)=reverse-scored item.

of psychopathy, antisocial behavior, substance use, empathy, and fear (Drislane et al. 2019).

PID-5 Forensic Faceted Brief Form

Because of the relevance of dysfunctional personality traits for predicting deviant behavior (Edens et al. 2015; Miller and Lynam 2001), Niemeyer et al. (2022) used the PID-5 Short Form (PID-5-SF) item pool to develop a psychometrically sound version of the PID-5-SF targeted to the forensic context, the PID-5 Forensic Faceted Brief Form (PID-5-FFBF). Niemeyer et al. (2022) aimed at capturing forensically relevant personality traits in order to provide clinicians information for forensic and correctional decision-making. With this aim, in a pilot study, Niemeyer et al. (2022) administered the PID-5-SF in a prison and collected 27 self-reports and 48 informant reports; the authors found acceptable psychometric properties for the PID-5-SF but observed some issues related to the poor fit of selected PID-5 items to the reality of life in prison. In particular, some PID-5-SF items were less relevant for incarcerated participants (e.g., "I often forget to pay my bills") or had a different literal meaning in the forensic context (e.g., "run away"); other items required clarification of the frame of reference (e.g., typical behavior or current life in prison, such as with the item "I'm not interested in making friends").

On the basis of the results of the pilot study, Niemeyer et al. (2022) adapted the PID-5-SF item content and developed the PID-5-FFBF, a 100-item self-report and informant report version of the PID-5-SF. With respect to the PID-5-SF, 18 items (20 for informant reports) were not adapted at all, 36 items were adapted to increase the fit of items to life in a prison setting, 34 items (32 for informant reports) were simplified in language, and 12 were slightly modified to focus on concrete rather than hypothetical behaviors. In line with the original PID-5, the PID-5-FFBF items are measured on a 4-point Likert-type scale ranging from 0 ("very false or often false") to 3 ("very true or often true"). PID-5-FFBF item content for the self-report and informant report versions of the measure can be found in Niemeyer et al.'s (2022) supplementary material (available at https://osf.io/p23t8).

Notably, Niemeyer et al. (2022) found adequate reliability for the PID-5-FFBF domain and trait scales; moreover, the PID-5-FFBF domains showed meaningful associations with the Five Factor Model traits and differential relationships, with indicators of psychological adjustment and forensically relevant constructs. As a whole, the PID-5-FFBF seemed to enable the assessment of dysfunctional personality traits in a forensic context.

Scoring Procedure for Malignant Narcissism Based on the PID-5

Recently, Faucher et al. (2022) developed a scoring procedure for malignant narcissism (i.e., narcissistic features intertwined with psychopathy/antisociality, sadism, paranoia, and aggressiveness; Lenzenweger et al. 2018) using the PID-5 trait scores. To this aim, Faucher et al. (2022) relied on a prototype matching approach, based on the ratings of specialists in personality disorder assessment and/or treatment. The resulting scoring procedure included 11 PID-5 facets; a weighting computation system allowed for reflecting the relative importance of each PID-5 trait (Faucher et al. 2022). Interestingly, a scoring sheet for "Malignant Narcissism Based on the PID-5" is provided as supplemental material for Faucher et al.'s (2022) study. The adequacy of this scoring procedure for clinical and research settings was assessed in a sample of clinical participants from a personality disorder treatment clinic, as well as in a sample of 1,103 participants from the community (Faucher et al. 2022).

CONCLUSION

The PID-5 scales and scoring methods briefly presented in this chapter suggest that this assessment instrument could be easily adapted to specific assessment needs. This flexibility makes it possible for both clinicians and researchers to think about the PID-5 as an assessment tool that could offer information about not only DSM-5 AMPD pathological personality traits but also other diagnostic models (e.g., ICD-11 personality domains) and forensic constructs (e.g., psychopathy). Future developments of the PID-5 scoring methods may meet other specific assessment needs (e.g., counterproductive work behavior and organizational citizenship behavior; Anderson 2022).

REFERENCES

American Psychiatric Association: Diagnostic and Statistical Manual of Mental Disorders, 5th Edition. Washington, DC, American Psychiatric Association, 2013

Anderson EL: Counterproductive work behavior and organizational citizenship behavior: understanding their nature and antecedents through familial, longitudinal, and concurrent data. Ph.D. dissertation, University of Minnesota, Minneapolis, 2022. [Dissertation Abstracts International: Section B: The Sciences and Engineering 84(2-B), 2022]

Bach B, Mulder R: Clinical implications of ICD-11 for diagnosing and treating personality disorders. Curr Psychiatry Rep 24(10):553–563, 2022a 36001221

Bach B, Mulder R: Empirical foundation of the ICD-11 classification of personality disorders, in Personality Disorders and Pathology: Integrating Clinical Assessment and Practice in the DSM-5 and ICD-11 Era. Edited by Huprich SK. Washington, DC, American Psychological Association, 2022b, pp 27–52

Bach B, Zine El Abiddine F: Empirical structure of DSM-5 and ICD-11 personality disorder traits in Arabic-speaking Algerian culture. Int J Ment Health 49:186–200, 2020

Bach B, Sellbom M, Kongerslev M, et al: Deriving ICD-11 personality disorder domains from DSM-5 traits: initial attempt to harmonize two diagnostic systems. Acta Psychiatr Scand 136(1):108–117, 2017 28504853

Bach B, Sellbom M, Skjernov M, et al: ICD-11 and DSM-5 personality trait domains capture categorical personality disorders: finding a common ground. Aust N Z J Psychiatry 52(5):425–434, 2018 28835108

Bach B, Kerber A, Aluja A, et al: International assessment of DSM-5 and ICD-11 personality disorder traits: toward a common nosology in DSM-5.1. Psychopathology 53(3–4):179–188, 2020 32369820

Crego C, Widiger TA: The convergent, discriminant, and structural relationship of the DAPP-BQ and SNAP with the ICD-11, DSM-5, and FFM trait models. Psychol Assess 32(1):18–28, 2020 31328932

Crego C, Samuel DB, Widiger TA: The FFOCI and other measures and models of OCPD. Assessment 22(2):135–151, 2015 24963102

Drislane LE, Sellbom M, Brislin SJ, et al: Improving characterization of psychopathy within the Diagnostic and Statistical Manual of Mental Disorders, Fifth Edition (DSM-5), Alternative Model for Personality Disorders: creation and validation of Personality Inventory for DSM-5 Triarchic scales. Personal Disord 10(6):511–523, 2019 31259604

Edens JF, Cox J, Smith ST, et al: How reliable are Psychopathy Checklist-Revised scores in Canadian criminal trials? A case law review. Psychol Assess 27(2):447–456, 2015 25486503

Fang S, Ouyang Z, Zhang P, et al: Personality Inventory for DSM-5 in China: evaluation of DSM-5 and ICD-11 trait structure and continuity with personality disorder types. Front Psychiatry 12:635214, 2021 33841206

Faucher J, Savard C, Vachon DD, et al: A scoring procedure for malignant narcissism based on Personality Inventory for DSM-5 facets. J Pers Assess 104(6):723–735, 2022 35025712

Hemmati A, Rahmani F, Bach B: The ICD-11 personality disorder trait model fits the Kurdish population better than the DSM-5 trait model. Front Psychiatry 12:635813, 2021 33859581

International Advisory Group for the Revision of ICD-10 Mental and Behavioural Disorders: A conceptual framework for the revision of the ICD-10 classification of mental and behavioural disorders. World Psychiatry 10(2):86–92, 2011 21633677

Kerber A, Schultze M, Müller S, et al: Development of a short and ICD-11 compatible measure for DSM-5 maladaptive personality traits using ant colony optimization algorithms. Assessment 29(3):467–487, 2022 33371717

Krueger RF, Derringer J, Markon KE, et al: Initial construction of a maladaptive personality trait model and inventory for DSM-5. Psychol Med 42(9):1879–1890, 2012 22153017

Lenzenweger MF, Clarkin JF, Caligor E, et al: Malignant narcissism in relation to clinical change in borderline personality disorder: an exploratory study. Psychopathology 51(5):318–325, 2018 30184541

Lotfi M, Bach B, Amini M, et al: Structure of DSM-5 and ICD-11 personality domains in Iranian community sample. Pers Ment Health 12(2):155–169, 2018 29392855

Lugo V, de Oliveira SES, Hessel CR, et al: Evaluation of DSM-5 and ICD-11 personality traits using the Personality Inventory for DSM-5 (PID-5) in a Brazilian sample of psychiatric inpatients. Pers Ment Health 13(1):24–39, 2019 30353698

McCabe GA, Widiger TA: A comprehensive comparison of the ICD-11 and DSM-5 Section III personality disorder models. Psychol Assess 32(1):72–84, 2020 31580095

Miller JD, Lynam D: Structural models of personality and their relation to antisocial behavior: a meta-analytic review. Criminology 39:765–798, 2001

Mulder RT, Newton-Howes G, Crawford MJ, et al: The central domains of personality pathology in psychiatric patients. J Pers Disord 25(3):364–377, 2011 21699397

Mulder RT, Horwood J, Tyrer P, et al: Validating the proposed ICD-11 domains. Personal Ment Health 10(2):84–95, 2016 27120419

Niemeyer LM, Grosz MP, Zimmermann J, et al: Assessing maladaptive personality in the forensic context: development and validation of the Personality Inventory for DSM-5 Forensic Faceted Brief Form (PID-5-FFBF). J Pers Assess 104(1):30–43, 2022 34037499

Oltmanns JR, Widiger TA: A self-report measure for the ICD-11 dimensional trait model proposal: the Personality Inventory for ICD-11. Psychol Assess 30(2):154–169, 2018 28230410

Patrick CJ, Drislane LE: Triarchic model of psychopathy: origins, operationalizations, and observed linkages with personality and general psychopathology. J Pers 83(6):627–643, 2015 25109906

Patrick CJ, Fowles DC, Krueger RF: Triarchic conceptualization of psychopathy: developmental origins of disinhibition, boldness, and meanness. Dev Psychopathol 21(3):913–938, 2009 19583890

Sellbom M, Solomon-Krakus S, Bach B, et al: Validation of Personality Inventory for DSM-5 (PID-5) algorithms to assess ICD-11 personality trait domains in a psychiatric sample. Psychol Assess 32(1):40–49, 2020 31204821

Somma A, Gialdi G, Fossati A: Reliability and construct validity of the Personality Inventory for ICD-11 (PiCD) in Italian adult participants. Psychol Assess 32(1):29–39, 2020 31414851

Tyrer P: Diagnostic and Statistical Manual of Mental Disorders: a classification of personality disorders that has had its day. Clin Psychol Psychother 19(5):372–374, 2012 22865543

Tyrer P, Crawford M, Mulder R, et al: The rationale for the reclassification of personality disorder in the 11th revision of the International Classification of Diseases (ICD-11). Pers Ment Health 5:246–259, 2011

Tyrer P, Reed GM, Crawford MJ: Classification, assessment, prevalence, and effect of personality disorder. Lancet 385(9969):717–726, 2015 25706217

Watters CA, Bagby RM: A meta-analysis of the five-factor internal structure of the Personality Inventory for DSM-5. Psychol Assess 30(9):1255–1260, 2018 29952594

Widiger TA, Simonsen E: Alternative dimensional models of personality disorder: finding a common ground. J Pers Disord 19(2):110–130, 2005 15899712

World Health Organization: ICD-11 Clinical Descriptions and Diagnostic Requirements for Mental and Behavioural Disorders. January 2023. Available at: https://icd.who.int/en. Accessed January 25, 2023.

CHAPTER 6

The PID-5 in Relationship With Other Measures

Since the publication of DSM-5 (American Psychiatric Association 2013), a number of studies have examined relationships between Personality Inventory for DSM-5 (PID-5) scales and measures of contemporary models of personality traits and psychopathology. This body of research aims to establish meaningful interconnections between models and measures that are routinely used in clinical practice and research contexts to assess personality and psychopathology. In this chapter, we provide clinicians and researchers with a summary of the main relationships between the PID-5 and widely used measures of personality and personality pathology. The ambition is to promote translation between well-established measures and models and the PID-5 and DSM-5 trait model to help clinicians and researchers who are very familiar with instruments commonly used across different applied contexts use the PID-5. Because this chapter does not represent an exhaustive presentation of the personality models, interested readers may refer to the cited works to obtain further details and information.

FIVE FACTOR MODEL MEASURES

As stated in DSM-5, the Alternative Model for Personality Disorders personality domains are "maladaptive variants of the five domains of the extensively validated and replicated personality model known as the 'Big Five', or Five Factor Model of personality" (American Psychiatric Association 2013, p. 773). The Five Factor Model (FFM) is a major dimensional model of personality (Widiger and Crego 2019) with roots in the Big Five lexical model (de Raad and Mlačić 2017). According to the lexical model, the structure of personality is reflected in natural language used to describe it, specifically in the empirical relationships among descriptors of personality (Allport 1937; Widiger and McCabe 2020). Research on the empirical structure of personality descriptors has pointed to five fundamental domains of personality: neuroticism (or negative emotionality vs. emotional stability; e.g., moody and anxious vs. calm and not easily upset), extraversion (or positive emotionality vs. introversion; e.g., talkative, assertive, and energetic vs. reserved and aloof), openness to experience (e.g., intellectual, curious, and creative vs. unimaginative and conventional); agreeableness (vs. antagonism or disagreeableness; e.g., cooperative and caring vs. hostile, aggressive, and callous), and conscientiousness (vs. disinhibition; e.g., orderly, responsible, and dependable vs. impulsive, disorganized, and unreliable). Notably, studies on the overlap between normative and maladaptive personality traits suggest that extreme variants of normative personality are maladaptive and associated with psychopathology and that pathological personality traits can be treated in the same framework as other personality traits (Markon et al. 2005; Widiger 2011).

Not surprisingly, since the publication of DSM-5, several empirical studies have examined relationships between PID-5 scales and different FFM measures. These studies have shown the convergence between PID-5 domains and FFM dimensions, relying on different FFM-based measures (e.g., the Five Factor Model Personality Disorder scales [Widiger et al. 2012], the International Personality Item Pool [Goldberg et al. 2006], NEO Personality Inventory-3 [McCrae et al. 2005]), different research methods (e.g., exploratory factor analysis, item response theory), and different samples (e.g., clinical, community) of different ages (i.e., adolescents, adults). This body of research suggests that with the partial exception of PID-5 psychoticism and openness to experience, PID-5 domains represent extreme variants of FFM dimensions at the phenotypic (e.g., Gore and Widiger 2013; Suzuki et al. 2015, 2017; Watson et al. 2013) and genetic (Wright et al. 2017) levels.

There may appear to be slight differences in the placement of selected PID-5 traits within the FFM; for instance, depressivity is treated as a facet of the PID-5 detachment domain, whereas it is treated as a facet of neuroticism within the FFM; similarly, suspiciousness is treated as a facet of PID-5 detachment, but it is a facet of antagonism according to the FFM (e.g., Widiger and McCabe 2020). These differences are often somewhat superficial, however, and can be explained by the multidimensionality of specific traits; PID-5 depressivity has relationships with both negative affect and detachment, even though it is more strongly related to the latter (Watters and Bagby 2018). Moreover, it should be observed that the FFM dimensions are bipolar: FFM measure scores often range from high levels of one pole (e.g., extraversion) to high levels of its opposite (e.g., introversion). In contrast, the PID-5 generally focuses on specific poles of the target traits (e.g., detachment or low extraversion), being designed to cover one extreme and maladaptive pole of a specific dimension (e.g., Krueger and Markon 2014; Suzuki et al. 2015).

Even keeping these differences in mind, available empirical evidence suggests that PID-5 traits and domains may be perceived as maladaptive, extreme variants of FFM facets and traits, and PID-5 dimensions could be conceptualized as instantiations of the FFM. Accordingly, clinicians and researchers may administer the PID-5 to obtain a precise assessment of personality traits, focusing on dysfunctional variants. Additionally, clinicians and researchers could interpret FFM measure scores in the light of their continuity with DSM-5 trait model dimensions and PID-5 scores as indexes of extreme variants of FFM traits (e.g., Suzuki et al. 2015).

MINNESOTA MULTIPHASIC PERSONALITY INVENTORY

Associations Between the PID-5 and the MMPI

The Minnesota Multiphasic Personality Inventory (MMPI) represents one of the most widely and frequently used psychopathology measures in clinical practice (e.g., Camara et al. 2000). Accordingly, examining the associations between the PID-5 and MMPI scales could establish important links between the two frameworks for assessing personality pathology. Sellbom et al. (2013) examined the association between the MMPI-2-Restructured Form (MMPI-2-RF) scales (Ben Porath and Tellegen 2011) and the PID-5 trait and domain scales in a large sample of more than 600 participants. The authors considered all MMPI-2-RF scales located across the three levels of its measurement hierarchy: the three Higher-Order scales representing broadband measures of psychopathology, the Restructured Clinical scales at the intermediate level, and the Specific Problems scales, which represent narrowband measures of facets associated with the Restructured Clinical scales. As a whole, Sellbom et al.'s (2013) findings supported convergence between the PID-5 domain and trait scale scores and the MMPI-2-RF scale scores, particularly at the domain level. For instance, MMPI-2-RF emotional-internalizing dysfunction, behavioral-externalizing dysfunction, and thought dysfunction were aligned with PID-5 negative affect and detachment, antagonism and disinhibition, and psychoticism, respectively.

As might be expected on the basis of the nature of their origins, no one-to-one correspondence was observed between PID-5 trait scales and MMPI-2-RF scales (Sellbom et al. 2013.) However, the two models generally converged at the more specific levels, with the large majority of the specific PID-5 traits being captured by MMPI-2-RF scales. For instance, the PID-5 Anxiousness scale showed significant relationship with the MMPI-2-RF Specific Problems Stress/Worry scale, PID-5 Anhedonia was associated with the MMPI-2-RF Low Positive Emotions scale, PID-5 Callousness was associated with the MMPI-2-RF Aggression scale, and PID-5 Distractibility was related to the MMPI-2-RF Cognitive Complaints scale (Sellbom et al. 2013).

Personality Psychopathology Five Domains

A five-factor dimensional model of personality is also assessed with the MMPI-2-RF. The MMPI-2-RF Personality Psychopathology Five (PSY-5) domains provide dimensional measures of personality pathology linking the MMPI-2-RF to a model of psychopathology focused on the FFM of personality (e.g., Widiger and Simonsen 2005). Given the conceptual links of the respective FFM traits and PSY-5 scales, it is not surprising that the DSM-5 domains, as assessed by the PID-5, showed substantial convergence with corresponding PSY-5 domains (Anderson et al. 2013). Indeed, the PSY-5 model describes dysfunctional personality dimensions according to five broad domains: namely, negative emotionality/neuroticism, introversion/low positive emotionality, aggressiveness, disconstraint, and psychoticism (Harkness and McNulty 1994). Specifically, the PSY-5 negative emotionality/neuroticism domain captures the disposition to experiencing a broad range of negative emotional experiences; thus, it is similar to FFM neuroticism and the PID-5 domain of negative affect. Introversion/low positive emotionality describes a lack of positive emotional experiences and avoidance of social situations. It describes introverted social detachment and low hedonic capacity, being akin to low FFM extraversion and PID-5 detachment. Aggressiveness measures aggressive behavior, including interpersonal dominance, callousness, grandiosity, and proclivity toward using instrumental aggression; it is akin to FFM low agreeableness and PID-5 antagonism. Disconstraint depicts a variety of manifestations of disinhibited behavior, comprising behavioral impulsivity and sensation seeking; accordingly, it is similar to FFM low conscientiousness and PID-5 disinhibition. Finally, PSY-5 psychoticism portrays a variety of experiences associated with thought disorder, including poor reality testing; thus, it is conceptually similar to PID-5 psychoticism, with some facets of FFM openness to experience (e.g., Ben Porath and Tellegen 2020).

Anderson et al. (2013) documented the convergence between the PSY-5 personality pathology model and the PID-5 domains in a sample of 463 undergraduate students. Correlation analysis and exploratory factor analysis results provided support for congruence between the PID-5 model and the PSY-5 model. Anderson et al.'s (2013) findings showed that the PSY-5 domains converge appropriately with PID-5 domains, supporting the usefulness of the PID-5 and the PSY-5 in assessing personality pathology. Because the DSM-5 Section III trait model considers personality disorders as characterized by specific configurations of traits, the lack of facet measurement in the PSY-5 scales makes it difficult to assign specific DSM-5 personality disorder diagnoses solely using these scales. However, like the PID-5—Brief Form (PID-5-BF) scores (see Chapter 3, "The PID-5s"), the PSY-5 domains can be used as a screening for general personality pathology (e.g., Anderson et al. 2013); they also can be used to support a given diagnosis whose differential assignment is based on other criteria.

PERSONALITY ASSESSMENT INVENTORY

Hopwood et al. (2013) examined the convergence of PID-5 traits with a sound and widespread dimensional measure of psychopathology, the Personality Assessment Inventory (PAI; Morey 1991). The PAI is a 344-item self-report instrument covering the constructs most relevant to a broad-based assessment of psychopathology (Morey 2007). The PAI has higher-order factors, including internalizing, externalizing, and social dominance (e.g., Hopwood and Moser 2011). These three factors were hypothesized to be linked to PID-5 negative affect, disinhibition, and low detachment, respectively. In their seminal study, Hopwood et al. (2013) administered both the 220-item PID-5 and the PAI in a sample of about 1,000 participants and found support for a substantial convergence of the two instruments.

The findings of Hopwood et al.'s (2013) study were important in suggesting the opportunity to adopt the PID-5 in those clinical and research contexts in which assessors are already familiar with and trained in the use of the PAI. Indeed, the joint structure of the PID-5 and PAI dimensions reflects broad psychological dimensions useful for identifying the relationships among personality, personality psychopathology, and clinically relevant behavior. Building on Hopwood et al.'s (2013) results, Busch et al. (2017) developed an initial strategy for using the PAI scores to explicitly assess DSM-5 dysfunctional personality traits, providing the opportunity to make inferences about personality and psychopathology constructs by relying on instruments that are widely used in many clinical settings.

SCHEDULE FOR NONADAPTIVE AND ADAPTIVE PERSONALITY

The Schedule for Nonadaptive and Adaptive Personality–Second Edition (SNAP-2; Clark et al. 2014) is a widely used 375-item true-false measure that assesses three broad temperament dimensions—namely, the Big Three (negative affectivity, positive affectivity, and disinhibition vs. constraint)—using 15 underlying personality facets (negative temperament, mistrust, manipulativeness, aggression, self-harm, eccentric perceptions, dependency, positive temperament, exhibitionism, entitlement, detachment, disinhibition, impulsivity, propriety, and workaholism). The SNAP-2 higher-order Big Three traits are theoretically connected to PID-5 dimensions—in particular, PID-5 negative affect with SNAP-2 negative temperament, PID-5 detachment with SNAP-2 positive temperament, and PID-5 disinhibition and antagonism with SNAP-2 disinhibition (e.g., Markon et al. 2005).

In their seminal study, Watson et al. (2013) examined the relationships between the PID-5 traits and the higher-order dimensions of the SNAP-2 in an outpatient sample of more than 200 patients and concluded that the PID-5 traits mapped onto SNAP-2 Big Three domains. The SNAP-2 and PID-5 higher-order dimensions jointly represent pathological variants of basic personality domains common to both pathological and nonpathological personality.

COMPUTERIZED ADAPTIVE TEST OF PERSONALITY DISORDER—STATIC FORM

The Computerized Adaptive Test of Personality Disorder—Static Form (CAT-PD-SF; Simms et al. 2011; Wright and Simms 2014) measures a comprehensive set of higher- and lower-order traits accounting for personality pathology. The CAT-PD model contains 33 lower-order scales organized into 5 higher-order domains consistent with the PSY-5 model (Harkness et al. 1995): negative emotionality, detachment, antagonism, disconstraint, and psychoticism. Wright and Simms (2014) examined the relationships between the PID-5 domains and the CAT-PD dimensions in a large clinical sample of outpatients and found a strong convergence between the CAT-PD and the PID-5 domains. These findings were replicated in an independent study conducted in a sample of 286 community adults undergoing mental health treatment or with a history of mental health treatment (Crego and Widiger 2016), as well as in subsequent research (Crego et al. 2018).

DIMENSIONAL ASSESSMENT OF PERSONALITY PATHOLOGY—BASIC QUESTIONNAIRE

The Dimensional Assessment of Personality Pathology—Basic Questionnaire (DAPP-BQ; Livesley and Jackson 2009) is a dimensional measure of personality pathology designed to assess personality disorders along the full continuum from mild to extreme trait manifestations. The DAPP-BQ items are grouped into 18 lower-order traits organized in four higher-order dimensions labeled as emotional dysregulation, inhibitedness, dissocial behavior, and compulsivity. As expected on the basis of theoretical considerations, empirical studies conducted in both community (e.g., Van den Broeck et al. 2013) and clinical (e.g., Bastiaens et al. 2016) participants showed that PID-5 negative affect, detachment, and antagonism domains were aligned with DAPP-BQ emotional dysregulation, inhibitedness, and dissocial dimensions, respectively.

CONCLUSION

As a whole, the PID-5 trait and domain scales have evinced theoretically meaningful and empirically significant overlap with a variety of widely used, sound measures of personality traits, many of which were developed according to different models of personality and personality pathology. This evidence suggests that PID-5 scores can be interpreted in the light of their continuities with other measures and models. Moreover, the findings briefly reviewed in this chapter suggest that the PID-5 instruments may be easily adopted by clinicians and researchers who are well acquainted with other measures. PID-5 dimensions showed significant associations with commonly adopted measures of personality and psychopathology, suggesting that they may easily interface with different models and instruments.

REFERENCES

Allport GW: Personality: A Psychological Interpretation. New York, Holt, 1937

American Psychiatric Association: Diagnostic and Statistical Manual of Mental Disorders, 5th Edition. Washington, DC, American Psychiatric Association, 2013

Anderson JL, Sellbom M, Bagby RM, et al: On the convergence between PSY-5 domains and PID-5 domains and facets: implications for assessment of DSM-5 personality traits. Assessment 20(3):286–294, 2013 23297369

Bastiaens T, Claes L, Smits D, et al: The construct validity of the Dutch Personality Inventory for DSM-5 Personality Disorders (PID-5) in a clinical sample. Assessment 23(1):42–51, 2016 25736039

Ben Porath YS, Tellegen A: Minnesota Multiphasic Personality Inventory-2 Restructured Form: Manual for Administration, Scoring, and Interpretation. Minneapolis, University of Minnesota Press, 2011

Ben Porath YS, Tellegen A: MMPI-3 Manual for Administration, Scoring and Interpretation. Minneapolis, University of Minnesota Press, 2020

Busch AJ, Morey LC, Hopwood CJ: Exploring the assessment of the DSM-5 Alternative Model for Personality Disorders with the Personality Assessment Inventory. J Pers Assess 99(2):211–218, 2017 27598924

Camara WJ, Nathan JS, Puente AE: Psychological test usage: implications in professional psychology. Prof Psychol Res Pr 31:141–154, 2000

Clark LA, Simms LJ, Wu KD, Casillas A: Manual for the Schedule for Nonadaptive and Adaptive Personality—2nd Edition (SNAP-2). Minneapolis, University of Minnesota Press, 2014

Crego C, Widiger TA: Convergent and discriminant validity of alternative measures of maladaptive personality traits. Psychol Assess 28(12):1561–1575, 2016 27046273

Crego C, Oltmanns JR, Widiger TA: FFMPD scales: comparisons with the FFM, PID-5, and CAT-PD-SF. Psychol Assess 30(1):62–73, 2018 29323514

de Raad B, Mlačić B: The lexical foundation of the Big Five factor model, in The Oxford Handbook of the Five Factor Model. Edited by Widiger TA. New York, Oxford University Press, 2017, pp 191–216

Goldberg LR, Johnson JA, Eber HW, et al: The International Personality Item Pool and the future of public-domain personality measures. J Res Pers 40:84–96, 2006

Gore WL, Widiger TA: The DSM-5 dimensional trait model and five-factor models of general personality. J Abnorm Psychol 122(3):816–821, 2013 23815395

Harkness AR, McNulty JL: The Personality Psychopathology Five (PSY-5): issue from the pages of a diagnostic manual instead of a dictionary, in Differentiating Normal and Abnormal Personality. Edited by Strack S, Lorr M. New York, Springer, 1994, pp 291–315

Harkness AR, McNulty JL, Ben-Porath YS: The Personality Psychopathology Five (PSY-5): constructs and MMPI-2 scales. Psychol Assess 7:104–114, 1995

Hopwood CJ, Moser JS: Personality Assessment Inventory internalizing and externalizing structure in college students: invariance across sex and ethnicity. Pers Individ Dif 50:116–119, 2011

Hopwood CJ, Wright AG, Krueger RF, et al: DSM-5 pathological personality traits and the Personality Assessment Inventory. Assessment 20(3):269–285, 2013 23610235

Krueger RF, Markon KE: The role of the DSM-5 personality trait model in moving toward a quantitative and empirically based approach to classifying personality and psychopathology. Annu Rev Clin Psychol 10:477–501, 2014 24329179

Livesley WJ, Jackson DN: Manual for the Dimensional Assessment of Personality Pathology—Basic Questionnaire (DAPP-BQ). Port Huron, MI, Sigma, 2009

Markon KE, Krueger RF, Watson D: Delineating the structure of normal and abnormal personality: an integrative hierarchical approach. J Pers Soc Psychol 88(1):139–157, 2005 15631580

McCrae RR, Costa PT Jr, Martin TA: The NEO-PI-3: a more readable revised NEO Personality Inventory. J Pers Assess 84(3):261–270, 2005 15907162

Morey LC: Professional Manual for the Personality Assessment Inventory. Odessa, FL, Psychological Assessment Resources, 1991

Morey LC: Professional Manual for the Personality Assessment Inventory, 2nd Edition. Lutz, FL, Psychological Assessment Resources, 2007

Sellbom M, Anderson JL, Bagby RM: Assessing DSM-5 Section III personality traits and disorders with the MMPI-2-RF. Assessment 20(6):709–722, 2013 24220212

Simms LJ, Goldberg LR, Roberts JE, et al: Computerized adaptive assessment of personality disorder: introducing the CAT-PD project. J Pers Assess 93(4):380–389, 2011 22804677

Suzuki T, Samuel DB, Pahlen S, et al: DSM-5 Alternative Personality Disorder Model traits as maladaptive extreme variants of the Five-Factor Model: an item-response theory analysis. J Abnorm Psychol 124(2):343–354, 2015 25665165

Suzuki T, Griffin SA, Samuel DB: Capturing the DSM-5 Alternative Personality Disorder Model traits in the Five-Factor Model's nomological net. J Pers 85(2):220–231, 2017 26691245

Van den Broeck J, Bastiaansen L, Rossi G, et al: Age-neutrality of the trait facets proposed for personality disorders in DSM-5: a DIFAS analysis of the PID-5. J Psychopathol Behav Assess 35:487–494, 2013

Watson D, Stasik SM, Ro E, et al: Integrating normal and pathological personality: relating the DSM-5 trait-dimensional model to general traits of personality. Assessment 20(3):312–326, 2013 23596272

Watters CA, Bagby RM: A meta-analysis of the five-factor internal structure of the Personality Inventory for DSM-5. Psychol Assess 30(9):1255–1260, 2018 29952594

Widiger T: Personality and psychopathology. World Psychiatry 10(2):103–106, 2011 21633679

Widiger TA, Crego C: The Five Factor Model of personality structure: an update. World Psychiatry 18(3):271–272, 2019 31496109

Widiger TA, McCabe GA: The Alternative Model of Personality Disorders (AMPD) from the perspective of the Five-Factor Model. Psychopathology 53(3–4):149–156, 2020 32526758

Widiger TA, Simonsen E: Alternative dimensional models of personality disorder: finding a common ground. J Pers Disord 19(2):110–130, 2005 15899712

Widiger TA, Lynam DR, Miller JD, et al: Measures to assess maladaptive variants of the Five-Factor Model. J Pers Assess 94(5):450–455, 2012 22519804

Wright AGC, Simms LJ: On the structure of personality disorder traits: conjoint analyses of the CAT-PD, PID-5, and NEO-PI-3 trait models. Pers Disord 5(1):43–54, 2014 24588061

Wright ZE, Pahlen S, Krueger RF: Genetic and environmental influences on Diagnostic and Statistical Manual of Mental Disorders-Fifth Edition (DSM-5) maladaptive personality traits and their connections with normative personality traits. J Abnorm Psychol 126(4):416–428, 2017 28368150

CHAPTER 7

Interpreting PID-5 Profiles

Comorbidity has been widely noted in the scientific literature on personality disorders, having been pointed to as a challenge to the validity and clinical utility of categorical approaches to personality disorder diagnosis (e.g., Clark 2007). The complexity of dysfunctional personality trait profiles observed across different clinical contexts accounts in part for the tendency to meet criteria for several personality disorder diagnoses simultaneously (e.g., Widiger and Trull 2007). The proposal made in the DSM-5 Alternative Model for Personality Disorders (AMPD; American Psychiatric Association 2013) allows clinicians to diagnose a single personality disorder whose specific features are tailored to the patient's problems. Describing the personality difficulties experienced by a person via their own trait profile is a methodologically sound approach to recognizing the richness of individual differences in the process of clinical decision-making.

From this point of view, Personality Inventory for DSM-5 (PID-5) domain scale scores might be seen as useful in pointing to the presence of clinically significant personality problems that manifest in multiple or more generalized ways, whereas PID-5 trait scores can be used to identify more specific problems that are more limited or narrower in scope. In this way, clinicians may rely on a two-part strategy for the clinical use of PID-5 scale score profiles, ignoring the often forced search for a match between the profile of a patient and the typological profile associated with a specific personality disorder diagnosis.

Although there are many ways to use the PID-5 in clinical assessment, at this time we suggest the following approach to clinical use and interpretation of a PID-5 profile:

1. Consider the PID-5 validity scale scores in combination with other sources of information about the validity of the test responses.
2. If these considerations indicate that the test responses are interpretable, consider the profiles of domain and trait scale scores. In doing this, remember that within the AMPD the use of the whole trait profile can be useful in obtaining a detailed description of personality problems without necessarily matching the profile to classical diagnostic prototypes.

Tables of T scores and percentiles corresponding to raw scores are given in the Appendix, "Normative Score Distributions." In the future, it may be possible to estimate the effect of response bias and inconsistency on trait estimates directly by incorporating validity scale and self- and informant ratings into trait and standard error estimates in a single step. This would likely be integrated in a software solution.

When using PID-5 profiles in clinical practice for the purpose of obtaining diagnoses according to the AMPD, the above two-step procedure should be used in tandem with an assessment of AMPD Criterion A (i.e., functioning) to arrive at a diagnostic decision. Assessment of Criterion A could be based on a few methods, such as a standardized interview-based assessment (e.g., using Module I of the Structured Clinical Interview for the DSM-5 Alternative Model for Personality Disorders [SCID-5-AMPD]; Bender et al. 2018) or other clinical assessment of Criterion A (e.g., Level of Personality Functioning Scale score; American Psychiatric Association 2013).

In this chapter, we consider the self-report and informant report versions of the PID-5. Individual profiles based on other versions of PID-5 (e.g., PID-5—Brief Form or PID-5—Short Form) might suggest other clinical interpretations.

CLINICAL EXAMPLES AND VIGNETTES

Mike

Mike, a 25-year-old man hospitalized in a general psychiatry department, works as a sound technician. He was hospitalized because he was no longer able to perform daily activities because of a sense of fatigue, weakness, and loss of interest. He also reported anxiety symptoms and panic attacks and has ruminative thoughts about the past. The psychiatrist in charge prescribed drug therapy with alprazolam, and during the hospitalization Mike asked for psychotherapy to manage his negative emotions.

During initial psychotherapy sessions, Mike had difficulty maintaining eye contact with the clinician. He told the psychologist that the onset of his symptoms could be traced back to a year before the hospitalization, when his girlfriend of 6 years ended their relationship. To manage his anxiety, Mike progressively started avoiding situations that might increase tension. Eventually, he was unable to leave home and was forced to quit working. Moreover, he explained, "I am unable to manage my own life," adding, "I am scared of assuming responsibilities and am terrified by the idea of reaching happiness and then losing it soon after." He believes that most of his anxiety is related to fear of abandonment and especially fear of losing his parents.

When asked about his relationships, Mike reported difficulties fitting in with peers since middle school. Specifically, he felt different from others and believed that he was the subject of ridicule. He described himself as shy and unable to interact with other people. In particular, he has always felt inferior compared with others. He told the clinician that he is always fearful and expects to be judged, criticized, and emotionally hurt. For these reasons, Mike admitted that he easily makes up stories, which he considers to be "impulsive."

In the past few years, Mike has generally avoided starting conversations with other people because, as he stated, "I feel observed when I talk; it has always been difficult for me to socialize." Mike explained that when he sees a group of people laughing, he believes that they are making fun of him. Furthermore, he described himself as a detached person who is not interested in other people's problems.

Despite having generally low self-regard, Mike said that he feels better when other people appreciate and admire him and feels miserable when other people do not recognize what he does. He compensates for this low self-esteem with fantasies of success and recognition from others (e.g., he dreams about becoming popular among his colleagues). Moreover, he daydreams about provoking pain in the people who have hurt him. Mike described feeling good about himself when he is "in a position of power and advantage over others."

Last, Mike highlighted a fear of being kidnapped and tortured and described himself as a suspicious person. Accordingly, he believes that he must keep an eye open to avoid feeling used by people he cannot trust. Because of this fear, he has interrupted some friendships in the past when those friendships became too close.

Description of Mike's PID-5 Profile

Table 7–1 provides Mike's scores on the PID-5 validity, domain, and trait scales.

Table 7–1. PID-5 validity, domain, and trait scales: Mike's scores

PID-5 scales	Raw score	T score
Validity		
VRIN	4	—
ORS	2	—
PRD	38	—
Domain		
Negative affect	2.68	82
Detachment	2.24	77–78
Antagonism	1.32	64–65
Disinhibition	2.38	87–88
Psychoticism	1.27	65–66
Trait		
Anxiousness	2.89	77–78
Emotional lability	2.43	73–74
Hostility	2.10	70–71
Perseveration	1.78	67–68
Restricted affectivity	1.43	59–60
Separation insecurity	2.71	81–82
Submissiveness	1.00	48–49
Anhedonia	3.00	86
Depressivity	2.79	93
Intimacy avoidance	0.83	54–55
Suspiciousness	2.00	70–71
Withdrawal	2.90	77–78
Manipulativeness	1.20	57–58
Deceitfulness	2.10	83–84
Grandiosity	0.67	49–50
Attention seeking	1.00	55
Callousness	1.00	65–66
Distractibility	3.00	84
Impulsivity	2.00	72–73
Rigid perfectionism	2.50	72–73

Table 7–1. PID-5 validity, domain, and trait scales: Mike's scores *(continued)*

PID-5 scales	Raw score	T score
Trait *(continued)*		
Risk taking	0.14	33–34
Irresponsibility	2.14	92–93
Eccentricity	1.85	66
Perceptual dysregulation	1.33	73
Unusual beliefs and experiences	0.63	52–53

Note. ORS=Over-Reporting Scale; PID-5=Personality Inventory for DSM-5; PRD= Positive Impression Management Response Distortion; VRIN=Variable Response Inconsistency.

On the basis of the PID-5 validity scales, Mike's PID-5 profile can be considered valid. Mike obtained a total raw score of 4 on the PID-5 Variable Response Inconsistency (PID-5-VRIN) scale, which suggests that Mike's responses to the PID-5 items were coherent and not random. Furthermore, the PID-5 Over-Reporting Scale (PID-5-ORS) score of 2 indicates that he likely was not exaggerating psychopathology. Last, the PID-5 Positive Impression Management Response Distortion (PID-5-PRD) score of 38 indicates that he likely was providing genuine responses. Figure 7–1 shows Mike's domain and trait profiles.

With regard to the PID-5 domain scales, Mike presented with significant elevations in the domains of negative affect (*T*=82), detachment (*T*=77–78), and disinhibition (*T*=87–88). His domain scale profile suggests the possibility of clinically significant problems, particularly in the areas of disinhibition, negative affect, and detachment.

The PID-5 trait profile suggests problems characterized by high neuroticism (i.e., negative affect). Specifically, Mike describes himself as prone to chronic nervousness, tension, or panic in reaction to different situations. At the same time, he experiences frequent worry about the negative effects of unpleasant past experiences and possible negative future events, as well as feelings of fear in new situations (high anxiousness; *T*=77–78). Additionally, Mike presents with a significant elevation on PID-5 separation insecurity (*T*=81–82) and describes himself as characterized by fear of being left alone because of rejection or separation from significant figures such as his parents. This may be related to a

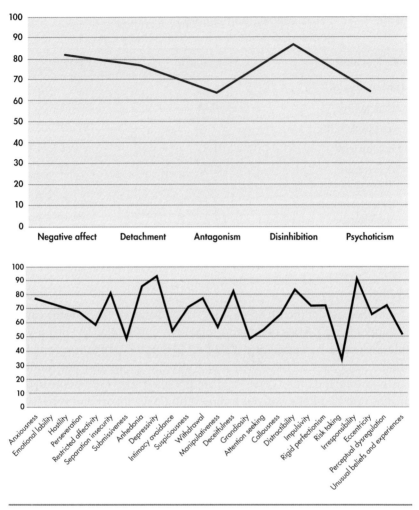

Figure 7–1. **Mike's Personality Inventory for DSM-5 domain (*top*) and trait (*bottom*) profiles.**

mistrust in his own capacity to take care of himself. Mike's trait profile is also characterized by persistent or frequent feelings of anger and irritability (hostility; $T=70–71$). This trait scale score could provide Mike's clinician with useful information in characterizing the aggressive fantasies reported by Mike during the clinical interview and how they might change with intervention.

Furthermore, Mike reports instability in his emotional experiences and that he perceives himself as prone to intense emotions that emerge easily and appear disproportionate to the event that has triggered them (emotional lability; $T=73-74$). His personality profile is characterized by withdrawal from interpersonal relationships and by a limited capacity to feel pleasure. Indeed, Mike describes himself as characterized by an inability to feel pleasure from life experiences and by a lack of interest in things (anhedonia; $T=86$). He reports constant feelings of discouragement, lack of hope, and pessimism for the future (depressivity; $T=93$). Moreover, he describes himself as a person showing sensitivity to malicious signs or interpersonal aggressiveness (suspiciousness; $T=70-71$) and a high preference for being alone rather than with other people, accompanied by avoidance of social contact and activities (withdrawal; $T=77-78$).

Mike also exhibits antagonist traits that manifest in a tendency to deceive in order to influence or control others or to obtain what he desires (deceitfulness; $T=83-84$). Moreover, Mike describes himself as an impulsive person inclined to act on a momentary basis without a plan (impulsivity; $T=72-73$). Mike also reports concentration difficulty, such as sustaining focus on tasks, with a consequent inability to produce a final product (distractibility; $T=84$), and lack of respect for agreements or promises (irresponsibility; $T=92-93$).

Mike's profile is informed also by an elevation in perceptual dysregulation ($T=73$), suggesting that Mike is inclined toward depersonalization and derealization and other unusual perceptual experiences, such as mixed sleep-wake states; this inclination toward dissociative experiences could be useful in understanding Mike's tendency to lose himself in fantasies. To conclude, Mike's PID-5 trait profile provides his clinician with a useful summary of his interpersonal style and difficulties, illustrating an active system of trait variables and their intensity.

Daniel

Daniel, a 27-year-old university student, asked for psychotherapy in an outpatient clinic. He reported anxiety, describing a tendency to ruminate on both positive and negative events. He also reported recurrent anger outbursts that he could not handle anymore. He asked for a psychological assessment, saying, "I want to name my suffering."

Daniel reported that he has "always felt bad" since he was 16 years old and has had problems with anger outbursts. During these episodes, Daniel loses control and is "unable to think." Moreover, on such occasions, he starts screaming and throwing objects. He also specified that these breakdowns often occur when other people do not meet his expectations or do not consider him as he would.

During initial interviews, it became clear that for Daniel, anxiety is also strongly related to anger. Indeed, the thoughts that Daniel finds himself ruminating about mostly concern past situations in which he feels that he has not received adequate acknowledgment or has been wronged. He talked about events that happened years before, and he reported that when he thinks about them, he still feels resentment. Daniel described himself as "very touchy," and over the course of his life, this has led him to end relationships with several friends.

Daniel also has anxiety problems related to his university studies. He is almost always worried about being able to achieve results that match the standards he has set for himself. He reported that even when he achieves success, such as a good grade on an important examination, he is unable to enjoy the moment; rather, he immediately starts setting even higher standards for subsequent assignments and repetitively wondering if he will be able to achieve them. Although Daniel described himself as "very ambitious and oriented toward achieving success and recognition," he does not have a very clear idea of what he would like to do once he finishes his studies.

In describing his relationships, Daniel reported that he has no significant relationships, with the partial exception of his family and a couple of friends. He said that he has difficulty maintaining romantic relationships because when the relationship begins to become intimate and his partner starts expressing "a very strong need for closeness," he breaks things off. He also described the fear of being left, and he usually suspects that his partner may lie to him or cheat on him. He acknowledged that the tendency to be distrustful of others has "always been part of my character" and has become an issue in several relationships, including those with the clinicians who treated him previously. Notwithstanding these difficulties, Daniel stated that he is "empathetic, sweet, and generous"; he also recognized that he is willing to help other people when he knows that being caring will result in gaining admiration or favors.

As for his childhood, Daniel described himself as a very irritable child and adolescent. He was often involved in physical fights with peers during childhood, and when he was a teenager, he damaged other people's property (e.g., keyed cars). Finally, he reported often using deception or lies to gain advantage, either for fun or from fear of being judged negatively.

Description of Daniel's PID-5 Profile

Table 7–2 lists Daniel's scores on the PID-5 validity, domain, and trait scales.

On the basis of the PID-5 validity scales, Daniel's profile appears to be valid. Daniel obtained a total score of 7 on the PID-5-VRIN scale, suggesting that his responses were coherent and not random. Furthermore, the PID-5-ORS score of 0 suggests no problem with exaggerating psychopathology. Last, the PID-5-PRD score of 27 seems to indicate a tendency

Table 7–2. PID-5 validity, domain, and trait scales: Daniel's scores

PID-5 scales	Raw score	T score
Validity		
VRIN	7	—
ORS	0	—
PRD	27	—
Domain		
Negative affect	2.31	75–76
Detachment	0.87	52
Antagonism	0.78	53–54
Disinhibition	1.89	77–78
Psychoticism	0.92	58–59
Trait		
Anxiousness	2.78	75–76
Emotional lability	2.71	77–78
Hostility	2.40	75
Perseveration	1.56	64–65
Restricted affectivity	0.00	30–34
Separation insecurity	1.43	61–62
Submissiveness	1.25	52–53
Anhedonia	1.50	61–62
Depressivity	1.36	66–67
Intimacy avoidance	0.50	49–50
Suspiciousness	2.43	77–78
Withdrawal	0.60	45–46
Manipulativeness	0.60	48–49
Deceitfulness	0.90	59–60
Grandiosity	0.83	52
Attention seeking	2.25	75
Callousness	0.71	58–59
Distractibility	2.56	77–78
Impulsivity	1.83	69–70
Rigid perfectionism	1.40	56–57

Table 7–2. PID-5 validity, domain, and trait scales: Daniel's scores *(continued)*

PID-5 scales	Raw score	*T* score
Trait *(continued)*		
Risk taking	1.64	62–63
Irresponsibility	1.29	72–73
Eccentricity	1.38	59–60
Perceptual dysregulation	0.75	59–60
Unusual beliefs and experiences	0.63	52–53

Note. ORS=Over-Reporting Scale; PID-5=Personality Inventory for DSM-5; PRD= Positive Impression Management Response Distortion; VRIN=Variable Response Inconsistency.

to give genuine responses, without obvious underreporting. Figure 7–2 shows Daniel's domain and trait profiles.

Daniel presented with significant elevations on the negative affect (*T*=75–76) and disinhibition (*T*=77–78) domains. This pattern of profile elevation is suggestive of clinically significant personality dysfunction.

On the PID-5 trait scales, Daniel describes himself as a person characterized by emotional instability manifesting in intense emotions that arise easily and may be disproportionate to events (high emotional lability; *T*=77–78). A significant PID-5 trait elevation was also observed for anxiousness (*T*=75–76), which is consistent with the reason for Daniel seeking a consultation. Not surprisingly, Daniel also described himself as experiencing persistent or frequent angry feelings in response to minor slights and insults (i.e., high hostility scores; *T*=75). In other words, Daniel perceives himself as a person characterized by feelings of nervousness, tension, or panic in reaction to different situations and by frequent worry about the negative effects of past unpleasant experiences and future negative events. He also sees himself as having difficulties with persistent and frequent feelings of anger, irritability in response to offenses and insults, and vengeful behavior.

At the same time, Daniel's PID-5 profile is characterized by an elevation on the Suspiciousness scale (*T*=77–78), suggestive of a tendency to be particularly sensitive to signs of malevolence or interpersonal aggression and to doubt the loyalty or faithfulness of others. In addition, Daniel's trait profile is characterized by high scores for attention seeking (*T*=75). In particular, Daniel describes himself as a person who car-

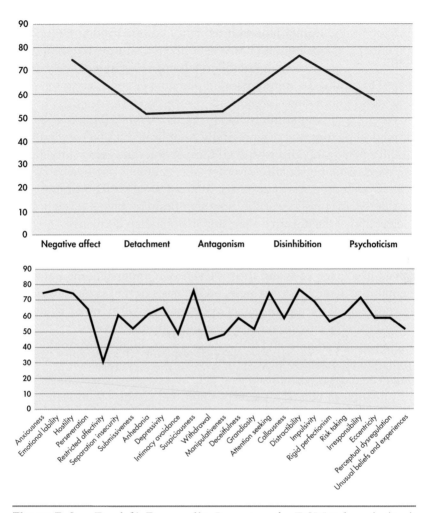

Figure 7–2. **Daniel's Personality Inventory for DSM-5 domain (*top*) and trait (*bottom*) profiles.**

ries out excessive attempts to gain attention and who seeks the admiration of others.

Notably, Daniel describes himself as a particularly distractible person with difficulty in maintaining purposeful behavior concerning both planning and task execution (high distractibility; $T=77–78$); moreover, he describes himself as characterized by a propensity toward disregarding his duties and being noncompliant with agreements and promises (irresponsibility; $T=72–73$). Daniel's trait profile is also characterized by borderline significant elevations ($66<T<71$) of other PID-5 facet scales, which may suggest the presence of a clinically relevant dysfunctionality. Specifically, Daniel reports a tendency toward feeling frequently sad, unhappy, hopeless, and pessimistic about the future (depressivity; $T=66–67$); he also describes himself as tending to act immediately in response to contingent stimuli without planning or considering the consequences of his actions (impulsivity; $T=69–70$).

When Daniel was administered the SCID-5-AMPD (First et al. 2016), the clinical picture was diagnostically complicated. Daniel met criteria for three personality disorder diagnoses—borderline personality disorder, narcissistic personality disorder, and paranoid personality disorder—as well as conduct disorder. When Daniel's PID-5 profile was considered, the presence of clinically significant problems was reflected in elevation of the negative affect and disinhibition domains.

The PID-5 trait profile helps clinicians obtain a fine-grained assessment of personality traits, providing a summary of different factors involved in a given case and their relevance in understanding patients' mental functioning. For example, on the basis of trait scale elevations, the most salient features of Daniel's personality style involve a tendency toward experiencing frequent worry about the negative effects of past unpleasant experiences and future negative possibilities. In addition, his emotional life seems to be governed by feelings of anger and irritability. Daniel also describes himself as a person actively engaged in seeking the attention of others, a predisposition that coexists with feelings of being mistreated, used, and persecuted by others. Distractibility also seems to be a particularly relevant characteristic of Daniel's personality.

Considering the patient's trait profile allows clinicians to adopt a more person-centered logic for the assessment of personality functioning, which allows them to capture 1) the different factors involved, 2) the patient's narrative profile in terms of how they tend to perceive and describe themselves, and 3) the interaction between maladaptive traits and the patient's life context.

Rick

Rick is a 55-year-old man without a permanent job, although he has done some occasional work as a truck driver. He asked for a clinical consultation for some behavioral problems that were putting his relationship with his partner at risk.

In the first interview, Rick talked about his decision to ask for help. This choice came after a suicide attempt triggered by his partner announcing that she was thinking about breaking up with him. The problems with his partner are related to frequent anger outbursts provoked by what he described as petty things. Rick reported that on these occasions he becomes verbally aggressive and yells things that he later regrets. Difficulties in managing anger have been a constant issue in his life. He also described that he has been reckless and impulsive since childhood. He reported a history of repeated unsafe sexual encounters, alcohol and substance use problems, and difficulties with management of his finances.

Rick's behavior seems to be strongly related to the context in which he lives. When he is in the "wrong crowd," he acts impulsively and sometimes illegally (e.g., dealing drugs). He also has had some difficulties in maintaining stable employment. However, he stated that when he was involved in relationships with "normal and respectable" women, his life was more stable, with fewer excesses.

Rick also talked about difficulties in maintaining stable relationships with friends and partners. His relationships usually ended because of his tendency to interpret others' behaviors in terms of unjustified offenses and injustices. Generally, he reacts to these situations in an aggressive way, including sometimes physically aggressive ways. He told the clinician that he needs "closeness in relationships," but at the same time, he reported that he is "not able to manage differences and disagreements," which makes his relationships particularly unstable.

Description of Rick's PID-5 Profile

Table 7–3 lists Rick's scores on the PID-5 validity, domain, and trait scales.

On the basis of the PID-5 validity scale scores, Rick's PID-5 domain and trait profile appear valid. He obtained a score of 6 on the PID-5-VRIN scale; this suggests that he was responding to items coherently and not responding randomly. Furthermore, the PID-5-ORS score suggests that he is not exaggerating psychopathology. Last, the PID-5-PRD scale score indicates that he was likely responding genuinely and was not portraying himself unrealistically. Figure 7–3 shows Rick's domain and trait profiles.

Rick presented with no significant elevation on PID-5 domains, with the partial exception of the domain of disinhibition ($T=67–68$), indicating a predisposition toward immediate gratification and impulsive behavior driven by current thoughts, feelings, and external stimuli, without regard to past experiences or consideration of future consequences. With regard to the PID-5 trait scales, Rick's profile is characterized by a tendency to experience feelings of persistent and frequent anger accompanied by irritability in response to insults or minor offenses (high hostility; $T=75$). The inclination toward hostility is associated with borderline elevated levels of suspiciousness ($T=67–68$). Rick describes himself as a person particularly responsive to signs of malevolence or interpersonal aggressiveness and to the feeling of being mis-

Table 7–3. PID-5 validity, domain, and trait scales: Rick's scores

PID-5 scales	Raw score	*T* score
Validity		
VRIN	6	—
ORS	1	—
PRD	21	—
Domain		
Negative affect	1.18	56–57
Detachment	0.37	42–43
Antagonism	0.86	55
Disinhibition	1.42	67–68
Psychoticism	0.00	35–40
Trait		
Anxiousness	0.67	46–47
Emotional lability	1.29	57
Hostility	2.40	75
Perseveration	0.33	43–44
Restricted affectivity	0.00	30–34
Separation insecurity	1.57	63–64
Submissiveness	0.00	30–33
Anhedonia	0.75	48–49
Depressivity	0.14	44–45
Intimacy avoidance	0.17	44–45
Suspiciousness	1.86	67–68
Withdrawal	0.20	39–40
Manipulativeness	0.80	51–52
Deceitfulness	1.10	63–64
Grandiosity	0.67	49–50
Attention seeking	1.25	59
Callousness	1.36	73–74
Distractibility	0.44	45–46
Impulsivity	2.67	83–84
Rigid perfectionism	0.00	30–35

Table 7–3. PID-5 validity, domain, and trait scales: Rick's scores *(continued)*

PID-5 scales	Raw score	*T* score
Trait *(continued)*		
Risk taking	2.29	75–76
Irresponsibility	1.14	69
Eccentricity	0.00	30–41
Perceptual dysregulation	0.00	30–42
Unusual beliefs and experiences	0.00	30–41

Note. ORS=Over-Reporting Scale; PID-5=Personality Inventory for DSM-5; PRD= Positive Impression Management Response Distortion; VRIN=Variable Response Inconsistency.

treated and used by other people. In addition, Rick's relational style is characterized by callousness (*T*=73–74); indeed, Rick describes himself as unable to worry about the feelings and problems of others and as someone who tends not to feel guilt or remorse for the negative effects of his own actions on others.

Rick's behavioral functioning is also reflected in elevations on the PID-5 trait scales of Impulsivity (*T*=83–84) and Risk Taking (*T*=75–76). Rick describes himself as acting immediately in response to contingent stimuli without planning or examining the consequences of his behavior and also as having difficulties in formulating or following plans. In addition, he describes himself as having a propensity to engage in activities that are dangerous, risky, and potentially harmful without necessity or concern for consequences. These elevations in impulsivity and risk taking scores are consistent with his elevated irresponsibility score (*T*=69) and are associated with irresponsible behaviors characterized by disinterest in honoring financial obligations or commitments and failure to honor and carry out agreements and promises.

Peter

Peter, a 33-year-old mechanic, asked for psychological consultation because of worsening psychological difficulties. He stated that the onset of the difficulties began about a year earlier, when "my insecurity became an obsession." He reported insomnia characterized by difficulties in falling asleep caused by ruminating over an assumed betrayal by his partner. Such thoughts made Peter excessively controlling of and "mor-

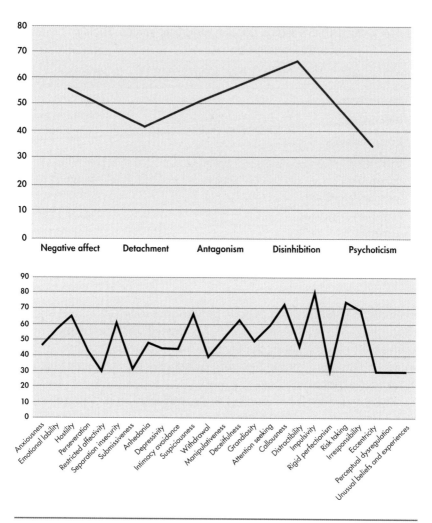

Figure 7–3.   Rick's Personality Inventory for DSM-5 domain (*top*) and trait (*bottom*) profiles.

bidly curious" about his girlfriend. Peter also reported feelings of being observed by unknown people, as if he were "at the center of the world." When he saw his neighbors interacting, he often thought that they were talking negatively about him. These thoughts became so pervasive that Peter decided to move because of the distress those ideas caused him. Peter sought psychological intervention in order to manage these thoughts, which have recently had a major effect on his life.

During the first assessment interview, Peter talked about the origin and development of his problems using vague, circumstantial, meta-phorical, and stereotypical speech. His problems with anxiety and depression made life difficult. In order to deal with them, he started avoiding situations. He abandoned his social life, which had a detrimental effect on his work performance. The depressive symptoms he reported included lack of energy and difficulties in dealing with the various commitments of daily life. Peter reported few friends throughout his life; even in the workplace, he did not establish any kind of close relationship with colleagues because of his lack of trust in others. He thinks that people judge him negatively and interact with him with malevolent intentions; he tends to perceive others as a potential source of threat. For these reasons, Peter has always preferred to be alone. He also reported difficulties in expressing and feeling emotions, describing himself as an "indifferent person," even in situations that other people would find engaging.

For the past few years, Peter has had a romantic relationship with a woman; this relationship has been characterized by distrust and anxiety. The fear of being betrayed led Peter to misinterpret his girlfriend's gestures, motivations, and behavior and to engage in controlling behavior toward her.

Peter also reported unusual experiences, such as feeling that an external force controls his thoughts and that a supernatural force "commands, controls, and makes things happen." He reported that he decided to buy a new car; specifically, on the suggestion of his boss, he opted to buy a green economy car. In the days following the decision, Peter reported that he continually came across this type of vehicle on the road, which he took as a sign that this was "the right car" for him. He also reported that he often has the feeling that objects in his house change position and that the presence of a "superior force" can explain such phenomena.

Detailed Description of Peter's PID-5 Profile

Table 7–4 provides Peter's scores on the PID-5 validity, domain, and trait scales.

On the basis of the PID-5 validity scales, Peter's PID-5 profile appears valid. He scored 9 on the PID-5-VRIN scale; this suggests that he was responding coherently. Furthermore, the PID-5-ORS score (equal to 0) suggests that psychopathological features conveyed by the PID-5 profile were not exaggerated. Finally, his PID-5-PRD score (37) suggests that he was being genuine in his responses and not underreporting. Figure 7–4 shows Peter's domain and trait scale scores.

With regard to the PID-5 domain scales, Peter presented with elevations on PID-5 psychoticism ($T=77-78$) and detachment ($T=75$). Consistent with his presentation in interview, he also had significantly elevated scores on PID-5 negative affect ($T=65-66$).

Table 7–4. PID-5 validity, domain, and trait scales: Peter's scores

PID-5 scales	Raw score	T score
Validity		
VRIN	9	—
ORS	0	—
PRD	37	—
Domain		
Negative affect	1.74	65–66
Detachment	2.10	75
Antagonism	0.71	51–52
Disinhibition	1.41	67–68
Psychoticism	1.90	77–78
Trait		
Anxiousness	1.56	58–59
Emotional lability	1.43	59
Hostility	2.03	69–70
Perseveration	1.22	58–59
Restricted affectivity	1.14	54–55
Separation insecurity	2.22	74
Submissiveness	1.71	58–59
Anhedonia	2.80	82–83
Depressivity	1.50	69–70
Intimacy avoidance	2.10	74–75
Suspiciousness	2.03	70–71
Withdrawal	1.40	56–57
Manipulativeness	0.80	51–52
Deceitfulness	1.00	61–62
Grandiosity	0.33	43–44
Attention seeking	1.31	60
Callousness	0.94	64
Distractibility	1.51	61–62
Impulsivity	1.35	61–62
Rigid perfectionism	1.20	53–54

Table 7–4. PID-5 validity, domain, and trait scales: Peter's scores *(continued)*

PID-5 scales	Raw score	*T* score
Trait *(continued)*		
Risk taking	1.80	65–66
Irresponsibility	1.36	74–75
Eccentricity	1.85	66
Perceptual dysregulation	1.75	82–83
Unusual beliefs and experiences	1.38	66–67

Note. ORS=Over-Reporting Scale; PID-5=Personality Inventory for DSM-5; PRD= Positive Impression Management Response Distortion; VRIN=Variable Response Inconsistency.

With regard to the PID-5 trait profile, Peter had the highest elevations in anhedonia (*T*=82–83) and perceptual dysregulation scores (*T*=82–83). Specifically, Peter described himself as a person unable to feel pleasure from experiences or to find energy for activities of life; moreover, he reported difficulty feeling pleasure and interest in things. A salient element of Peter's personality scale profile is the tendency to have thought processes that are bizarre or unusual and weird sensations across different sensorial modalities, accompanied by vague, circumstantial, and metaphorical speaking or thinking. Despite his concerns about distrust in interpersonal relationships, Peter scored only above average on suspiciousness (*T*=70–71) and hostility (*T*=69–70). However, his scores on intimacy avoidance (*T*=74–75) and separation insecurity (*T*=74) were both significantly elevated. These elevations are consistent with his reports in interview, which suggest that Peter tends to avoid intimate or affective relationships and fears rejection or separation from significant figures, excessive dependence, and complete loss of autonomy (separation insecurity; *T*=74). On the basis of these trait elevations, it appears that Peter oscillates between social withdrawal and the need for intense close relationships in which he may become suspicious and controlling. Together with his difficulty in taking pleasure in life, Peter is prone to feelings of discouragement, unhappiness, and hopelessness; pessimism toward the future; and experiences of pervasive shame and guilt (depressivity; *T*=69–70). Finally, his trait scale scores highlight possible problems with disinterest in and failure to honor and follow through on agreements and promises (irresponsibility; *T*=74–75).

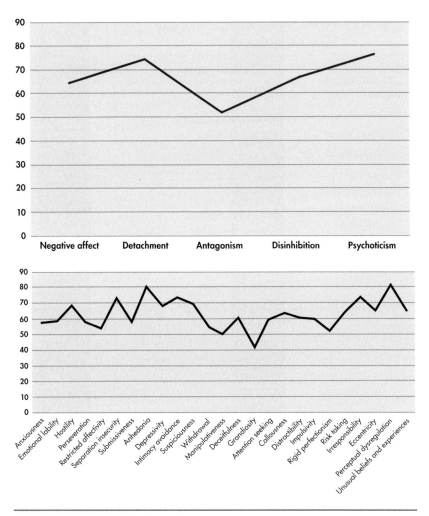

Figure 7–4.   Peter's Personality Inventory for DSM-5 domain (*top*) and trait (*bottom*) profiles.

USING THE PID-5—INFORMANT FORM IN CLINICAL PRACTICE

Although self-report measures play a central role in the assessment of personality pathology in clinical and research settings, there are situations in which informant report measures are critically valuable (see also Chapter 3, "The PID-5s," and Chapter 4, "PID-5 Response Validity Assessment and Validity Scales"). Informant reports offer a different source of information on the person being evaluated, which can be used to increase the validity and generalizability of conclusions. The PID-5—Informant Form (PID-5-IRF) provides informant report measures that parallel the PID-5 self-report in content and structure, which facilitates integration of measurements across sources. The PID-5-IRF is a useful measure in a number of scenarios, such as when additional sources of information are desired, when informant measures are expected to provide incremental validity over self-report, when relationships and social perception are a focal interest, and when response bias is a salient concern (e.g., Markon et al. 2013).

Maria

Maria, a 27-year-old programmer, sought services at a clinical psychology unit because of her low self-esteem and fear of being judged by others. These issues were causing her significant distress and "blocked" her across different situations.

During the interview, Maria reported that she has always had problems interacting with her peers and that she had only two friends during her high school years. She told clinicians that these friends are the most important persons in her life because they know her very well. Maria often experiences feelings of tension in relating to others because she is afraid of negative judgment. She reported that she had two significant romantic relationships; both ended because of her constant tendency to compare herself negatively with other people. Her partners were eventually exhausted by her behavior.

Maria attended a math and science academy for high school even though she would have preferred to pursue arts. The choice of the school was not because of her interests but rather because of the proximity of the school to her home. At the time of the interview, she was in a bachelor's degree program in design; however, her university career was hindered by very intense anxiety. Maria asked for help from the clinic when her anxiety was interfering significantly with her work on a final degree project (e.g., she was unable to write).

When talking about her family, Maria reported problems with her parents. In particular, she described her father as a man who is "difficult to understand" and is reserved and unwilling to express emotions. Despite these difficulties, she has managed to build a close relationship with him. Maria described her mother as "distant" and emotionally aloof. She described her relationship with her younger sister as difficult as well. Maria said that she constantly compares herself with her sister and believes that she will never be able to obtain the same confidence and personal fulfillment as her sister, who is married and expecting a child.

At the end of the first interview, the clinician asked Maria whether she would complete a self-report measure (the PID-5). Maria told the clinician that she preferred to have one of her friends complete the PID-

5-IRF because she was worried that she would not be able to respond accurately and that her responses would be too influenced by her fear of being judged.

Description of Maria's PID-5-IRF Profile

Table 7–5 provides Maria's scores on the PID-5-IRF domain and trait scales. Figure 7–5 shows Maria's domain and trait scale scores.

According to the PID-5-IRF, Maria presented with an above average elevation on the PID-5 Negative Affect domain scale (T=70–71), suggesting that others perceive her as experiencing clinically significant levels of a wide range of negative emotions (e.g., anxiety, depression, guilt/shame, worry, anger) and their interpersonal manifestations (e.g., dependency).

Consistent with her presentation in interview, Maria was described on the PID-5-IRF as having problems adapting her behavior to other people's interests and real and presumed desires, even when this is antithetical to her own interests, needs, and desires (i.e., submissiveness; T=75–76). In addition, Maria's profile was characterized by a perceived tendency to experience frequent feelings of nervousness, tension, or panic in reaction to different situations and to experience frequent worry about the negative effects of past unpleasant experiences and future negative events, along with feelings of fear and apprehension in situations of uncertainty by anticipating the worst (high anxiousness; T=82–83). Maria's trait profile also includes a significant elevation on emotional lability (T=71). This suggests that she is seen as being unstable in her emotional experiences and mood and indicates a tendency to experience intense emotions that arise easily and are often out of proportion to events and circumstances.

In summary, Maria's personality profile, at least as described by the PID-5-IRF, seems to indicate a specific significant area of personality impairment that mainly concerns high and unstable levels of negative emotion. Maria is seen by others as experiencing intense negative emotions such as anxiety and depression, which, at the interpersonal level, manifest in difficulties being assertive and independent. Her friend's ratings on the PID-5-IRF confirm Maria's presentation in interview, pointing to areas to address in therapy.

Lucy

Lucy, a 19-year-old undergraduate student, arrived at the clinic accompanied by her mother. She was unenthusiastic about receiving psychological treatment, but her mother thought it was necessary because of

Table 7–5. PID-5-IRF domain and trait scales: Maria's scores

PID-5-IRF scales	Raw score	T score
Domain		
Negative affect	2.12	70–71
Detachment	0.53	45–46
Antagonism	0.17	41–42
Disinhibition	0.79	52–53
Psychoticism	0.62	54–55
Trait		
Anxiousness	3.29	82–83
Emotional lability	2.43	71
Hostility	0.82	49–50
Perseveration	0.72	49–50
Restricted affectivity	1.28	54–55
Separation insecurity	0.65	48–49
Submissiveness	2.75	75–76
Anhedonia	1.25	56–57
Depressivity	0.71	53–54
Intimacy avoidance	0.00	30–40
Suspiciousness	0.43	43–44
Withdrawal	0.33	43–44
Manipulativeness	0.28	41–42
Deceitfulness	0.22	45
Grandiosity	0.00	30–41
Attention seeking	0.88	49–50
Callousness	0.00	30–41
Distractibility	0.73	50–51
Impulsivity	0.82	50
Rigid perfectionism	1.47	56–57
Risk taking	0.80	44–45
Irresponsibility	0.81	56–57
Eccentricity	1.09	56–57

Table 7–5. PID-5-IRF domain and trait scales: Maria's scores *(continued)*

PID-5-IRF scales	Raw score	*T* score
Trait *(continued)*		
Perceptual dysregulation	0.47	54
Unusual beliefs and experiences	0.30	50–51

Note. PID-5-IRF=Personality Inventory for DSM-5—Informant Form.

self-harm and anger-related problems. Lucy disclosed self-injury problems, and her mother explained that Lucy sometimes is verbally aggressive with family members. When Lucy becomes anxious or when emotions are experienced as "too strong" and unmanageable, she cuts her arms and legs. Lucy's mother explained that when Lucy gets angry, she is unable to control herself and becomes verbally abusive and insulting.

Lucy's mother reported that when Lucy was in primary school, her teachers were worried because "she would start crying, screaming, and throwing herself on the ground," abruptly and without any apparent explanation. When Lucy was 6 years old, she began to perform certain rituals (e.g., repeating phrases and numbers) to avoid bad consequences. Relatively quickly, these behaviors became more frequent and concerning, and as a result, Lucy's mother took her to a child psychiatrist. Lucy received a diagnosis of obsessive-compulsive disorder, which was treated with medication and cognitive-behavioral therapy. At age 14, Lucy started to have problems with food, alternating between fasting and binge eating. Moreover, she experienced difficulties in calming down when upset; Lucy's mother described her daughter as "always tense and grumpy." When Lucy was 17 years old, she started cutting herself to "calm down and be in touch with reality"; she also started consuming alcohol until drunk. On some occasions, she was able to ask for help when she was upset, and her mother was able to calm her down. Lucy described her mother as the "only person who can understand me," although they sometimes have "uncontrolled arguments." Lucy has a few close friends, but she is not able to talk with them about her problems. She reported feeling criticized all the time, as if every aspect of her life was under scrutiny by others: "The judgments affect everything…what I say, my physical appearance; I always need someone to reassure me." Indeed, Lucy is very interested in her friends' opinion: "If they don't consider me, I feel bad. Sometimes I get drunk so they pay attention to me." In addition, Lucy reported being very frightened because of unusual vivid daydreams. She started experiencing these daydreams in the past few weeks and has similar experiences almost every night before falling asleep.

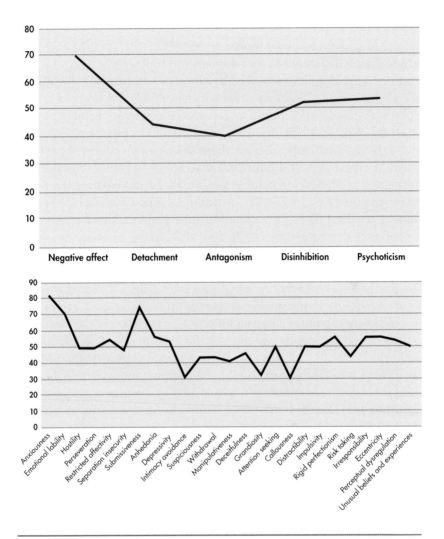

Figure 7–5. **Maria's Personality Inventory for DSM-5—Informant Form domain (*top*) and trait (*bottom*) profiles.**

After the first consultation, Lucy and her mother were asked to complete the self-report form of the PID-5 (PID-5-SRF) and PID-5-IRF, respectively. Lucy's PID-5-VRIN score of 20 suggested that she was responding incoherently to the PID-5-SRF. Because this score seemed to suggest that Lucy may have answered some PID-5-SRF questions inconsistently or randomly, the clinician decided to consider Lucy's PID-5-IRF profile instead.

Description of Lucy's PID-5-IRF Profile

Table 7–6 provides Lucy's scores on the PID-5-IRF domain and trait scales. Figure 7–6 shows Lucy's domain and trait scale scores.

Lucy's profile is characterized by elevations in scores on the PID-5-IRF Disinhibition ($T=73$) and Psychoticism ($T=75–76$) domain scales. Lucy was described as prone to experiencing intense feelings of nervousness, tension, or panic, often in reaction to interpersonal stresses, and as being constantly worried about the negative effects of past unpleasant experiences and future negative events, together with feelings of fear and apprehension in uncertain situations, anticipating the worst (high anxiousness; $T=78–79$). In addition, Lucy was rated by her mother on the PID-5-IRF as tending to experience intense, unstable emotions with frequent mood changes and having emotions that tend to arise easily, are intense, and often are disproportionate to the events and circumstances that triggered them (high emotional lability; $T=78–79$). Furthermore, another putative feature of Lucy's personality is extreme sensitivity in interpersonal relationships, as indexed by her fear of rejection or separation from significant figures, along with fears of excessive dependence and complete loss of autonomy (high separation insecurity; $T=79–80$). She was also rated as having a propensity to adapt her behavior to other people's real or presumed interests and desires, even when this was antithetical to her own interests and desires (high submissiveness scale; $T=78–79$). In addition, Lucy seems to be perceived as persisting in a particular activity or way of doing things much longer than is functional or effective by continuing in the same behavior despite numerous failures (high perseveration; $T=76–77$).

Simultaneous elevations of Depressivity ($T=85–86$) and Anhedonia ($T=71$) trait scale scores emerged from Lucy's PID-5-IRF trait profile. Such elevations are suggestive of the tendency to frequently feel sad, unhappy, and hopeless, with difficulty in recovering from these states. These traits are also characterized by thoughts of suicide and suicidal behavior (high depressivity) and an inability to derive enjoyment from life's experiences and to find the energy to cope with the various situations of daily life (high anhedonia). Research has suggested that this pattern of elevations (i.e., high depressivity and anhedonia), together with high scores on the Anxiousness scale, may be suggestive of suicidal risk in younger individuals (Somma et al. 2016) and may provide useful clinical indications for treatment planning. Together with the reported concerns in interview, Lucy's profile suggests the need for monitoring suicide risk over time. Moreover, significant trait profile el-

Table 7–6. PID-5-IRF domain and trait scales: Lucy's scores

PID-5-IRF scales	Raw score	*T* score
Domain		
Negative affect	2.00	68–69
Detachment	1.35	60
Antagonism	0.30	43–44
Disinhibition	2.01	73
Psychoticism	1.61	75–76
Trait		
Anxiousness	3.00	78–79
Emotional lability	3.00	78–79
Hostility	1.90	62–63
Perseveration	2.56	76–77
Restricted affectivity	0.14	37
Separation insecurity	2.86	79–80
Submissiveness	3.00	78–79
Anhedonia	2.25	71
Depressivity	2.71	85–86
Intimacy avoidance	1.00	54–55
Suspiciousness	1.86	65–66
Withdrawal	0.80	49–50
Manipulativeness	0.00	30–37
Deceitfulness	0.90	55–56
Grandiosity	0.00	30–41
Attention seeking	1.25	54–55
Callousness	0.00	30–41
Distractibility	2.56	77
Impulsivity	2.90	78–79
Rigid perfectionism	2.90	75–76
Risk taking	2.14	67–68
Irresponsibility	0.57	52
Eccentricity	1.43	61

Table 7–6. PID-5-IRF domain and trait scales: Lucy's
scores *(continued)*

PID-5-IRF scales	Raw score	*T* score
Trait *(continued)*		
Perceptual dysregulation	2.67	104
Unusual beliefs and experiences	0.74	60

Note. PID-5-IRF=Personality Inventory for DSM-5—Informant Form.

evations emerged in both PID-5-IRF Impulsivity (T=78–79) and Distractibility (T=77) scale scores, along with elevations in the Rigid Perfectionism scale score (T=75–76). These elevations seem to be suggestive of Lucy's tendency to experience episodes of both lack of control (i.e., acting on the spur of the moment and on a momentary basis without plan or consideration of outcomes, while experiencing difficulty in maintaining goal-focused behavior) and hypercontrol, as suggested by high scores on rigid perfectionism (i.e., rigid insistence on everything being flawless, perfect, and without errors or faults, including her performance). Consistent with Lucy's description, loss of control may manifest in the form of a sense of urgency and self-injurious behavior when she is subjected to emotional stress. Notably, Lucy's trait profile is also characterized by the presence of clinically relevant elevations of the PID-5-IRF Perceptual Dysregulation (T=104) scale; her mother described Lucy as prone to experiences of depersonalization and derealization and to experiences of mixed sleep-wake states. This pattern may be related to her self-injury and may be seen as a crucial aspect for treatment planning because of the need to assess and monitor Lucy's suicidal risk.

CONCLUSION

Many of the considerations that apply to the clinical interpretation of PID-5 domain and trait scale profiles apply to the clinical interpretation of any test score. Test interpretation should not be considered as a simple and mechanical procedure. An accurate test interpretation requires not only relying on a sound test provided with sound norms but also considering the characteristics of the person and the scenario. Clinical decision-making should be grounded in sound psychological mea-

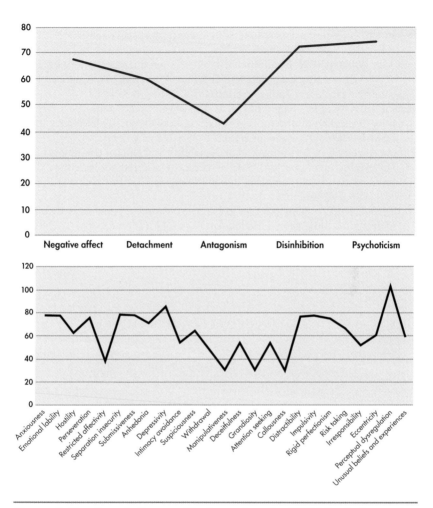

Figure 7–6. **Lucy's Personality Inventory for DSM-5—Informant Form domain (*top*) and trait (*bottom*) profiles.**

sures; clinicians should integrate test results with other considerations in the general assessment of the patient, taking into account the clinical context in which the psychological assessment took place.

REFERENCES

American Psychiatric Association: Diagnostic and Statistical Manual of Mental Disorders, 5th Edition. Washington, DC, American Psychiatric Association, 2013
Bender DS, Skodol AE, First MB, et al: Structured Clinical Interview for the DSM-5 Alternative Model for Personality Disorders (SCID-5-AMPD) Module I. Washington, DC, American Psychiatric Association Publishing, 2018

Clark LA: Assessment and diagnosis of personality disorder: perennial issues and an emerging reconceptualization. Annu Rev Psychol 58:227–257, 2007 16903806

First MB, Williams JBW, Benjamin LS, et al: Structured Clinical Interview for DSM-5 Personality Disorders (SCID-5-PD). Arlington, VA, American Psychiatric Association Publishing, 2016

Markon KE, Quilty LC, Bagby RM, et al: The development and psychometric properties of an informant-report form of the Personality Inventory for DSM-5 (PID-5). Assessment 20(3):370–383, 2013 23612961

Somma A, Fossati A, Terrinoni A, et al: Reliability and clinical usefulness of the Personality Inventory for DSM-5 in clinically referred adolescents: a preliminary report in a sample of Italian inpatients. Compr Psychiatry 70:141–151, 2016 27624434

Widiger TA, Trull TJ: Plate tectonics in the classification of personality disorder: shifting to a dimensional model. Am Psychol 62(2):71–83, 2007 17324033

CHAPTER 8

Prevention and Intervention

As has been emphasized throughout this book, the Personality Inventory for DSM-5 (PID-5; American Psychiatric Association 2013) approach to personality assessment allows clinicians to focus attention on a patient's unique personality profile rather than forcing their attention on how to place that profile into arbitrary categories. With the assessment process, this approach helps the clinician focus on a patient's unique circumstances and experiences; this in turn helps the clinician think about identifying the best treatment for that specific patient's unique problems. Scientific evidence provides consistent support for the general efficacy of psychotherapy for many mental disorders, with patient, clinician, and therapeutic relationship characteristics playing a role in psychotherapy outcome. The PID-5 helps identify some of the patient characteristics that might play a role in psychotherapy outcomes and how they might manifest in therapeutic and other relationships.

Although research in this area is developing, we believe that PID-5 profiles may provide a valuable tool for clinicians in their effort to identify the best treatment strategies for their patients. Moreover, assessments that use the PID-5 inherently encourage clinicians and their patients to take a psychological perspective in describing, and hopefully understanding, problematic intraindividual processes. This perspective is likely to help the clinician avoid a flight into medical jargon, medicalization, and superficial approaches to problems; it may move the patient's and clinician's orientation instead toward processes involved in the genesis and maintenance of problems and how to change those processes—that is, toward psychological mindedness and acceptance. Being rooted in basic personality theory as well as a transtheoretical approach to diagnosis, the PID-5 is an empirically based instrument that clinicians of different theoretical backgrounds can rely on in assessing an individual's personality profile to provide them with the best treatment options. The PID-5 dimensional approach may fit clinicians' attempts to create a shared perspective with patients in which psychotherapy is an interpersonal process aimed at promoting change rather an attempt at superficially eliminating symptoms of a medical syndrome or disease.

Psychological treatments with proven efficacy exist for numerous psychological disorders (e.g., Barlow 1996a), and patient variables, including personality traits and co-occurring symptoms, predict effects of psychological interventions (e.g., Barlow 1996b). Indeed, an impressive amount of data supporting evidence of clinical efficacy for several psychotherapies, both manualized and nonmanualized, led to the inclusion of empirically supported psychotherapy treatment in the clinical guidelines for treatment of several different disorders (e.g., Barlow 1996b). At the same time, a major change in the approach to designing and delivering psychotherapy, based on a dimensional perspective on psychopathology, has developed in the past 20 years (e.g., Barlow et al. 2017; Maples-Keller et al. 2019; Ruggero et al. 2019). Lack of empirical support for categorical approaches to mental disorders and the related need for psychotherapy approaches taking into account multiple, co-occurring diagnoses and symptoms have led researchers from very different theoretical backgrounds—for example, Barlow et al. (2011a, 2011b) from a cognitive-behavioral perspective and Leichsenring and Steinert (2018) from a psychodynamic perspective—to develop new empirically supported psychotherapy methods that are explicitly designed to target psychopathology dimensions common to a range of syndromes.

Personality traits are quintessential examples of such dimensions. Personality variables constitute core elements of psychopathology classification and structure when viewed from a dimensional perspective (Kotov et al. 2017) and have significant psychosocial relevance. Cuijpers et al. (2010) convincingly demonstrated that the personality dimension of neuroticism, at least in its extreme manifestations (which correspond to the PID-5 negative affect domain; American Psychiatric Association

2013; Suzuki et al. 2015), incurs economic costs exceeding those of common mental disorders (e.g., mood disorders, anxiety disorders, substance use disorders, somatic disorder), representing an impressive socioeconomic burden. Accordingly, Cuijpers et al. (2010) suggested thinking about psychological interventions that focus on the trait neuroticism rather than its specific outcomes. Similar points have been made by many other authors (e.g., Bleidorn et al. 2019; McAdams and Pals 2006).

A significant literature on interventions targeting personality variables, including pharmacological as well as psychotherapy interventions and their outcomes, has developed. Roberts et al. (2017) examined this literature meta-analytically, concluding that such interventions are effective for all trait domains across a range of settings, methods, and modalities, within time frames that are realistic for clinical practice. They noted that traits related to negative affect and detachment show the greatest changes when using existing interventions. Interventions are most effective in producing personality change among individuals with anxiety and personality disorder diagnoses and least effective among those with eating and substance use disorder diagnoses. Pharmacological and psychotherapy interventions of different modalities are all effective, with hospitalization-based approaches being least effective in changing personality variables. Given these findings, the PID-5 should be useful in planning and prioritizing goals for therapy and intervention, especially when considered as part of a broader psychiatric or medical evaluation.

It is important to consider prominent objections to the use of personality variables in therapy planning and practice—namely, that psychotherapy is neither suited to nor concerned with personality traits. Typically, reluctance to focus on personality variables in treatment and intervention follows from one of two common beliefs: 1) that personality traits are relatively fixed, unchanging features of a person and 2) that personality variables merely summarize more basic psychological processes that are themselves causally relevant. The first of these assumptions, as has been shown, is false in that personality does change and is changeable with intervention (e.g., Roberts et al. 2017). The second is a more substantive argument but, we believe, also misguided. For instance, this same literature on intervention and personality change suggests that intervention theories aimed at personality variables do result in meaningful, consequential change, supporting the role of personality variables as viable therapy goals. Moreover, even if personality variables are summaries of more specific psychological processes, those specific processes do cluster in predictable, replicable, transdiagnostic patterns (Kotov et al. 2017), and personality measures are effective indicators of those clusters. As such, from a predictive, informational view, assessment and therapeutic planning around personality variables are likely to be useful clinically and more broadly in policy (e.g., Bleidorn et al. 2019; McAdams and Pals 2006; Ruggero et al. 2019).

A substantial body of empirical research, which in part constituted the foundation of the DSM-5 Alternative Model for Personality Disorders (AMPD), suggests that PID-5 dimensions are likely to convey a large amount of therapy-relevant clinical information, which is not limited to the description of specific regulatory cognitive, affective, and motivational processes. For example, studies have indicated that PID-5 traits and domains show differential meaningful associations with adult attachment styles (e.g., Fossati et al. 2015), mentalization measures (e.g., Ball Cooper et al. 2021; Fossati et al. 2017), and a wide array of impairments in the areas of self- and interpersonal functioning (AMPD Criterion A; e.g., Nysaeter et al. 2023; Sleep and Lynam 2022). The PID-5 does not simply operationalize the DSM-5 AMPD Criterion B assessment; it gives expression via the assessment process to the AMPD ambition to provide clinicians with a way to link the stylistic (i.e., personality profile) with general impairment in personality functioning (e.g., self- and interpersonal functioning), both of which have consistently been noted to be cornerstones of clinical decision-making (e.g., Parker et al. 2004).

REFERENCES

American Psychiatric Association: Diagnostic and Statistical Manual of Mental Disorders, 5th Edition. Washington, DC, American Psychiatric Association, 2013

Ball Cooper E, Anderson JL, Sharp C, et al: Attachment, mentalization, and Criterion B of the Alternative DSM-5 Model for Personality Disorders (AMPD). Borderline Personal Disord Emot Dysregul 8(1):23, 2021 34334129

Barlow DH: The effectiveness of psychotherapy: science and policy. Clin Psychol 3:236–240, 1996a

Barlow DH: Health care policy, psychotherapy research, and the future of psychotherapy. Am Psychol 51(10):1050–1058, 1996b 8870541

Barlow DH, Ellard KK, Fairholme CP, et al: The Unified Protocol for Transdiagnostic Treatment of Emotional Disorders: Client Workbook. New York, Oxford University Press, 2011a

Barlow DH, Farchione TJ, Fairholme CP, et al: The Unified Protocol for Transdiagnostic Treatment of Emotional Disorders: Therapist Guide. New York, Oxford University Press, 2011b

Barlow DH, Farchione TJ, Bullis JR, et al: The unified protocol for transdiagnostic treatment of emotional disorders compared with diagnosis-specific protocols for anxiety disorders: a randomized clinical trial. JAMA Psychiatry 74(9):875–884, 2017 28768327

Bleidorn W, Hill PL, Back MD, et al: The policy relevance of personality traits. Am Psychol 74(9):1056–1067, 2019 31829685

Cuijpers P, Smit F, Penninx BW, et al: Economic costs of neuroticism: a population-based study. Arch Gen Psychiatry 67(10):1086–1093, 2010 20921124

Fossati A, Krueger RF, Markon KE, et al: The DSM-5 Alternative Model of Personality Disorders from the perspective of adult attachment: a study in community-dwelling adults. J Nerv Ment Dis 203(4):252–258, 2015 25756706

Fossati A, Somma A, Krueger RF, et al: On the relationships between DSM-5 dysfunctional personality traits and social cognition deficits: a study in a sample of consecutively admitted Italian psychotherapy patients. Clin Psychol Psychother 24(6):1421–1434, 2017 28493518

Kotov R, Krueger RF, Watson D, et al: The Hierarchical Taxonomy of Psychopathology (HiTOP): a dimensional alternative to traditional nosologies. J Abnorm Psychol 126(4):454–477, 2017 28333488

Leichsenring F, Steinert C: Towards an evidence-based unified psychodynamic protocol for emotional disorders. J Affect Disord 232:400–416, 2018 29522960

Maples-Keller JL, Yasinski C, Coghlan C, et al: Treatment of antagonism: cognitive behavioral therapy, in The Handbook of Antagonism. Edited by Miller JD, Lynam DR. Cambridge, MA, Academic Press, 2019, pp 351–364

McAdams DP, Pals JL: A new Big Five: fundamental principles for an integrative science of personality. Am Psychol 61(3):204–217, 2006 16594837

Nysaeter TE, Hummelen B, Christensen TB, et al: The incremental utility of Criteria A and B of the DSM-5 Alternative Model for Personality Disorders for predicting DSM-IV/DSM-5 Section II personality disorders. J Pers Assess 105(1):111–120, 2023 35285763

Parker G, Hadzi-Pavlovic D, Both L, et al: Measuring disordered personality functioning: to love and to work reprised. Acta Psychiatr Scand 110(3):230–239, 2004 15283744

Roberts BW, Luo J, Briley DA, et al: A systematic review of personality trait change through intervention. Psychol Bull 143(2):117–141, 2017 28054797

Ruggero CJ, Kotov R, Hopwood CJ, et al: Integrating the Hierarchical Taxonomy of Psychopathology (HiTOP) into clinical practice. J Consult Clin Psychol 87(12):1069–1084, 2019 31724426

Sleep CE, Lynam DR: The problems with Criterion A: a comment on Morey et al. (2022). Personal Disord 13(4):325–327, 2022 35787114

Suzuki T, Samuel DB, Pahlen S, et al: DSM-5 Alternative Personality Disorder Model traits as maladaptive extreme variants of the five-factor model: an item-response theory analysis. J Abnorm Psychol 124(2):343–354, 2015 25665165

APPENDIX

Normative Score Distributions

BACKGROUND AND METHODS

Norms for selected Personality Inventory for DSM-5 (PID-5; American Psychiatric Association 2013) scores (validity, domain, and trait scale scores for the 220-item and 100-item self-report form and the informant report form and the total score and domain scores for the brief form) and their differences are reported in Tables A–1 to A–12. Norms for the 220-item and 100-item forms and the brief form were obtained from a sample of 1,082 individuals from a U.S. Census–matched panel (Krueger et al. 2012). This is the same panel reported in the original PID-5 development article (Krueger et al. 2012), although the sample is different. Details regarding the sampling methodology and recruitment of participants are described in that article (Krueger et al. 2012). Norms for the informant form were derived from a sample of 360 individuals from the same panel, as described in detail by Markon et al. (2013). The differences in *T* scores reported in Table A–12 are based on a sample of 40 individuals who completed the self-report form and were rated by an informant (Markon et al. 2013).

Normative distributions for the self-report form validity scales were obtained from the entire sample of 1,082 individuals. Normative distributions for the self-report domain and trait scales were obtained from the subset of respondents who met the following inclusion criteria: their

PID-5 Variable Response Inconsistency (VRIN) scale scores were lower than 17, no more than a quarter of their responses were missing, and they did not endorse both infrequency items. This resulted in a sample size of 995 for the self-report form total score and domain and trait score datasets.

All self-report form descriptive statistics, T scores, and percentiles were computed using sampling weights reflecting U.S. Census data. Weights were not used with values involving the informant form because weights were not available for the subset of 40 participants nominated by a self-report respondent. Weights were not available for these participants because of uncertainty about whether to compute weights for the target, rater, or pair relative to weights for other participants who were sampled directly from the panel. Participants without weights were retained when calculating normative score distributions because all of the informant data samples were obtained via the Census-matched panel directly or indirectly and because dropping a subset of participants would decrease variation in the ways informants were recruited into participation relative to the targets of their ratings and the panel.

With weighting, 52% of the full self-report sample identified as female and the remaining 48% identified as male (unweighted summaries of demographic variables were similar; weighted values are reported for consistency with the score distribution estimates). Participants' ages ranged from 18 to 92, and the mean and median ages were 46.6 and 47 years, respectively. In terms of education, 11.5% completed less than a high school degree, 29.6% completed high school or equivalent, 28.3% reported having some college, and 30.7% reported having a bachelor's degree or higher. Of the sample, 67% identified as White, 11.7% as Black, 5.3% as other non-Hispanic, 14.7% as Hispanic, and 1.3% as more than one race. In terms of residence, 18.2% resided in the Northeast, 21.8% in the Midwest, 36.9% in the South, and 23.1% in the West; 16.1% resided in a nonmetropolitan region, and the remainder resided in a metropolitan region.

Without weighting, 52.5% of the informant report sample identified as female and 47.5% identified as male. Ages ranged from 19 to 93, and the mean and median ages were 50.4 and 53, respectively. In terms of education, 12.8% completed less than a high school degree, 25.8% completed high school or equivalent, 29.4% completed some college, and 31.9% completed a bachelor's degrees or higher. Of the sample, 73.9% identified as White, 10.8% as Black, 1.7% as other non-Hispanic, 11.4% as Hispanic, and 2.2% as more than one race. In terms of residence, 15.3% resided in the Northeast, 21.7% resided in the Midwest, 41.9% resided in the South, and 21.1% resided in the West; 19.4% resided in a nonmetropolitan region, and the remainder resided in a metropolitan region.

RESOURCES

The PID-5 is a freely available, American Psychiatric Association–approved instrument that can be employed easily by researchers and clinicians. The PID-5 items and scoring instructions for computing PID-5 domain and trait scales can be downloaded at www.psychiatry.org/psychiatrists/practice/dsm/educational-resources/assessment-measures#section_10.

The PID-5 can be reproduced, either electronically or in print formats, without permission by researchers and by clinicians solely for use with their patients in private practice, research, or hospital settings. In addition to the tables presented here, a computerized administration and scoring system that provides raw scores, *T* scores, and percentiles for the PID-5 scales is available at https://pid5-us-en.pegasopoint.it.

Table A–1. Personality Inventory for DSM-5—Self-Report Form Variable Response Inconsistency (VRIN) scale score percentiles

VRIN scale score	Percentile
0	0.03
1	0.06
2	0.09
3	0.13
4	0.20
5	0.30
6	0.38
7	0.48
8	0.55
9	0.63
10	0.72
11	0.78
12	0.83
13	0.87
14	0.90
15	0.93
16	0.94
17	0.95
18	0.97
19	0.98
20	0.99
21	0.99
22	0.99
23	1.00

Table A–2. Personality Inventory for DSM-5—Self-Report Form (100-item form) Variable Response Inconsistency (VRIN) scale score percentiles

VRIN scale score	Percentile
0	0.078
1	0.151
2	0.302
3	0.478
4	0.619
5	0.770
6	0.856
7	0.914
8	0.945
9	0.964
10	0.979
11	0.982
12	0.994
13	0.996
14	0.996
15	1.000

Table A–3. Personality Inventory for DSM-5—Self-Report Form Over-Reporting Scale score percentiles

Score	Percentile
0	0.889
1	0.974
2	0.993
3	0.996
4	0.999
5	0.999
6	0.999
7	0.999
8	1.000

Table A–4. Personality Inventory for DSM-5—Self-Report Form
Positive Impression Management Response Distortion
scale (underreporting) score percentiles

Score	Percentile
0	0.007
1	0.017
2	0.031
3	0.062
4	0.127
5	0.216
6	0.283
7	0.358
8	0.451
9	0.529
10	0.569
11	0.611
12	0.665
13	0.701
14	0.750
15	0.780
16	0.802
17	0.822
18	0.847
19	0.855
20	0.875
21	0.894
22	0.908
23	0.920
24	0.924
25	0.931
26	0.933
27	0.940
28	0.947
29	0.959

Table A–4. Personality Inventory for DSM-5—Self-Report Form Positive Impression Management Response Distortion scale (underreporting) score percentiles *(continued)*

Score	Percentile
30	0.971
31	0.979
32	0.981
33	0.982
34	0.984
35	0.984
36	0.984
37	0.988
38	0.989
39	0.990
40	0.990
41	0.992
42	0.993
43	0.994
44	0.998
45	0.998
46	0.998
47	0.998
48	0.998
49	0.999
50	0.999
51	0.999
52	0.999
53	0.999
54	0.999
55	1.000

Table A–5. Personality Inventory for DSM-5—Self-Report Form normative tables: domain scales

T	Negative affect		Detachment		Antagonism		Disinhibition		Psychoticism	
	Raw	Percentile	Raw	Percentile	Raw	Percentile	Raw	Percentile	Raw	Percentile
35	0.00	0.00	0.00	0.00	0.00	0.00	0.00	0.00	0.00	0.00
36	0.00	0.00	0.02	0.01	0.00	0.00	0.00	0.00	0.00	0.00
37	0.05	0.02	0.07	0.05	0.01	0.04	0.00	0.00	0.00	0.00
38	0.11	0.04	0.12	0.08	0.05	0.05	0.00	0.05	0.00	0.00
39	0.17	0.10	0.18	0.12	0.10	0.10	0.05	0.07	0.00	0.00
40	0.23	0.16	0.23	0.16	0.15	0.14	0.10	0.12	0.00	0.00
41	0.28	0.21	0.28	0.20	0.20	0.19	0.15	0.17	0.05	0.14
42	0.34	0.25	0.34	0.25	0.25	0.25	0.20	0.22	0.10	0.22
43	0.40	0.29	0.39	0.29	0.29	0.29	0.24	0.28	0.15	0.30
44	0.46	0.35	0.45	0.33	0.34	0.32	0.29	0.32	0.20	0.38
45	0.52	0.39	0.50	0.36	0.39	0.37	0.34	0.39	0.25	0.43
46	0.58	0.42	0.55	0.42	0.44	0.44	0.39	0.43	0.30	0.48
47	0.64	0.46	0.61	0.47	0.48	0.47	0.44	0.47	0.35	0.52
48	0.69	0.50	0.66	0.50	0.53	0.51	0.48	0.52	0.40	0.56
49	0.75	0.53	0.71	0.53	0.58	0.55	0.53	0.57	0.45	0.59
50	0.81	0.56	0.77	0.56	0.63	0.57	0.58	0.60	0.50	0.62

Table A–5. Personality Inventory for DSM-5—Self-Report Form normative tables: domain scales *(continued)*

T	Negative affect		Detachment		Antagonism		Disinhibition		Psychoticism	
	Raw	Percentile	Raw	Percentile	Raw	Percentile	Raw	Percentile	Raw	Percentile
51	0.87	0.61	0.82	0.59	0.67	0.59	0.63	0.64	0.55	0.65
52	0.93	0.64	0.87	0.63	0.72	0.63	0.68	0.68	0.60	0.67
53	0.99	0.68	0.93	0.67	0.77	0.66	0.73	0.71	0.65	0.70
54	1.04	0.71	0.98	0.70	0.82	0.69	0.77	0.73	0.70	0.73
55	1.10	0.74	1.03	0.72	0.86	0.72	0.82	0.75	0.75	0.75
56	1.16	0.77	1.09	0.75	0.91	0.75	0.87	0.77	0.80	0.77
57	1.22	0.79	1.14	0.78	0.96	0.78	0.92	0.78	0.85	0.79
58	1.28	0.81	1.19	0.80	1.01	0.80	0.97	0.81	0.90	0.81
59	1.34	0.82	1.25	0.82	1.06	0.83	1.01	0.83	0.95	0.82
60	1.40	0.84	1.30	0.82	1.10	0.85	1.06	0.85	1.00	0.83
61	1.45	0.85	1.35	0.84	1.15	0.86	1.11	0.86	1.05	0.84
62	1.51	0.87	1.41	0.85	1.20	0.88	1.16	0.87	1.10	0.86
63	1.57	0.88	1.46	0.87	1.25	0.90	1.21	0.89	1.16	0.88
64	1.63	0.89	1.51	0.89	1.29	0.91	1.25	0.90	1.21	0.89
65	1.69	0.90	1.57	0.91	1.34	0.92	1.30	0.91	1.26	0.90
66	1.75	0.91	1.62	0.92	1.39	0.92	1.35	0.93	1.31	0.92

Table A–5. Personality Inventory for DSM-5—Self-Report Form normative tables: domain scales *(continued)*

T	Negative affect		Detachment		Antagonism		Disinhibition		Psychoticism	
	Raw	Percentile	Raw	Percentile	Raw	Percentile	Raw	Percentile	Raw	Percentile
67	1.81	0.93	1.67	0.94	1.44	0.93	1.40	0.93	1.36	0.92
68	1.86	0.93	1.73	0.95	1.48	0.93	1.45	0.94	1.41	0.93
69	1.92	0.94	1.78	0.96	1.53	0.95	1.50	0.94	1.46	0.94
70	1.98	0.94	1.83	0.97	1.58	0.95	1.54	0.95	1.51	0.94
71	2.04	0.96	1.89	0.97	1.63	0.97	1.59	0.96	1.56	0.95
72	2.10	0.96	1.94	0.97	1.68	0.97	1.64	0.96	1.61	0.96
73	2.16	0.97	1.99	0.98	1.72	0.98	1.69	0.97	1.66	0.96
74	2.22	0.98	2.05	0.98	1.77	0.98	1.74	0.97	1.71	0.97
75	2.27	0.98	2.10	0.98	1.82	0.98	1.78	0.97	1.76	0.97
76	2.33	0.98	2.15	0.98	1.87	0.98	1.83	0.98	1.81	0.97
77	2.39	0.98	2.21	0.99	1.91	0.98	1.88	0.98	1.86	0.98
78	2.45	0.99	2.26	0.99	1.96	0.98	1.93	0.98	1.91	0.98
79	2.51	0.99	2.31	0.99	2.01	0.98	1.98	0.99	1.96	0.98
80	2.57	1.00	2.37	0.99	2.06	0.99	2.02	0.99	2.01	0.99
81	2.63	1.00	2.42	0.99	2.10	0.99	2.07	0.99	2.06	0.99
82	2.68	1.00	2.47	1.00	2.15	0.99	2.12	0.99	2.11	0.99

Table A–5. Personality Inventory for DSM-5—Self-Report Form normative tables: domain scales *(continued)*

T	Negative affect		Detachment		Antagonism		Disinhibition		Psychoticism	
	Raw	Percentile	Raw	Percentile	Raw	Percentile	Raw	Percentile	Raw	Percentile
83	2.74	1.00	2.53	1.00	2.20	0.99	2.17	0.99	2.16	0.99
84	2.80	1.00	2.58	1.00	2.25	1.00	2.22	0.99	2.21	1.00
85	2.86	1.00	2.63	1.00	2.29	1.00	2.27	0.99	2.26	1.00
86	2.92	1.00	2.69	1.00	2.34	1.00	2.31	0.99	2.31	1.00
87	2.98	1.00	2.74	1.00	2.39	1.00	2.36	0.99	2.36	1.00
88	3.04	1.00	2.79	1.00	2.44	1.00	2.41	1.00	2.41	1.00
89	3.09	1.00	2.85	1.00	2.49	1.00	2.46	1.00	2.46	1.00
90	3.15	1.00	2.90	1.00	2.53	1.00	2.51	1.00	2.51	1.00

Table A–6. Personality Inventory for DSM-5—Self-Report Form normative tables: trait scales

T	Anhedonia		Anxiousness		Attention seeking		Callousness		Deceitfulness	
	Raw	Percentile	Raw	Percentile	Raw	Percentile	Raw	Percentile	Raw	Percentile
30	0.00	0.00	0.00	0.00	0.00	0.00	0.00	0.00	0.00	0.00
31	0.00	0.00	0.00	0.00	0.00	0.00	0.00	0.00	0.00	0.00
32	0.00	0.00	0.00	0.00	0.00	0.00	0.00	0.00	0.00	0.00
33	0.00	0.00	0.00	0.00	0.00	0.00	0.00	0.00	0.00	0.00
34	0.00	0.00	0.00	0.00	0.00	0.00	0.00	0.00	0.00	0.00
35	0.00	0.00	0.00	0.00	0.00	0.00	0.00	0.00	0.00	0.00
36	0.00	0.00	0.00	0.00	0.00	0.00	0.00	0.00	0.00	0.00
37	0.05	0.05	0.00	0.00	0.00	0.00	0.00	0.00	0.00	0.00
38	0.11	0.05	0.06	0.04	0.00	0.00	0.00	0.00	0.00	0.00
39	0.17	0.11	0.14	0.13	0.00	0.00	0.00	0.00	0.00	0.00
40	0.23	0.11	0.21	0.13	0.06	0.19	0.00	0.00	0.00	0.00
41	0.29	0.19	0.28	0.19	0.12	0.19	0.00	0.00	0.01	0.22
42	0.35	0.19	0.35	0.29	0.18	0.28	0.01	0.20	0.05	0.22
43	0.41	0.29	0.42	0.29	0.25	0.28	0.05	0.20	0.10	0.34
44	0.47	0.30	0.50	0.36	0.31	0.38	0.09	0.34	0.15	0.34
45	0.53	0.42	0.57	0.43	0.37	0.38	0.13	0.34	0.20	0.46

Table A–6. Personality Inventory for DSM-5—Self-Report Form normative tables: trait scales *(continued)*

T	Anhedonia		Anxiousness		Attention seeking		Callousness		Deceitfulness	
	Raw	Percentile	Raw	Percentile	Raw	Percentile	Raw	Percentile	Raw	Percentile
46	0.59	0.42	0.64	0.43	0.43	0.46	0.18	0.46	0.25	0.46
47	0.65	0.50	0.71	0.49	0.50	0.46	0.22	0.56	0.30	0.46
48	0.71	0.50	0.79	0.54	0.56	0.53	0.26	0.57	0.35	0.55
49	0.77	0.56	0.86	0.54	0.62	0.53	0.30	0.63	0.40	0.56
50	0.83	0.56	0.93	0.58	0.68	0.58	0.35	0.63	0.45	0.62
51	0.89	0.64	1.00	0.63	0.75	0.58	0.39	0.70	0.50	0.62
52	0.95	0.64	1.07	0.63	0.81	0.62	0.43	0.75	0.54	0.69
53	1.01	0.72	1.15	0.67	0.87	0.62	0.47	0.76	0.59	0.69
54	1.07	0.72	1.22	0.67	0.94	0.68	0.52	0.79	0.64	0.74
55	1.13	0.76	1.29	0.71	1.00	0.68	0.56	0.80	0.69	0.74
56	1.19	0.76	1.36	0.74	1.06	0.73	0.60	0.83	0.74	0.78
57	1.25	0.79	1.43	0.75	1.12	0.73	0.64	0.84	0.79	0.79
58	1.31	0.80	1.51	0.78	1.19	0.78	0.69	0.84	0.84	0.83
59	1.37	0.80	1.58	0.80	1.25	0.78	0.73	0.86	0.89	0.83
60	1.43	0.84	1.65	0.80	1.31	0.81	0.77	0.86	0.94	0.86
61	1.49	0.84	1.72	0.84	1.37	0.81	0.81	0.88	0.99	0.86

Table A–6. Personality Inventory for DSM-5—Self-Report Form normative tables: trait scales *(continued)*

T	Anhedonia		Anxiousness		Attention seeking		Callousness		Deceitfulness	
	Raw	Percentile	Raw	Percentile	Raw	Percentile	Raw	Percentile	Raw	Percentile
62	1.55	0.86	1.79	0.86	1.44	0.86	0.86	0.88	1.03	0.89
63	1.61	0.86	1.87	0.86	1.50	0.89	0.90	0.91	1.08	0.89
64	1.67	0.89	1.94	0.88	1.56	0.89	0.94	0.92	1.13	0.92
65	1.73	0.89	2.01	0.90	1.63	0.92	0.98	0.92	1.18	0.92
66	1.79	0.93	2.08	0.90	1.69	0.92	1.03	0.93	1.23	0.93
67	1.85	0.93	2.16	0.92	1.75	0.94	1.07	0.93	1.28	0.93
68	1.92	0.94	2.23	0.94	1.81	0.94	1.11	0.94	1.33	0.94
69	1.98	0.94	2.30	0.94	1.88	0.97	1.15	0.95	1.38	0.94
70	2.04	0.95	2.37	0.96	1.94	0.97	1.20	0.95	1.43	0.94
71	2.10	0.95	2.44	0.96	2.00	0.98	1.24	0.95	1.47	0.95
72	2.16	0.96	2.52	0.97	2.06	0.98	1.28	0.95	1.52	0.96
73	2.22	0.96	2.59	0.98	2.13	0.98	1.32	0.95	1.57	0.96
74	2.28	0.98	2.66	0.98	2.19	0.98	1.37	0.96	1.62	0.96
75	2.34	0.98	2.73	0.98	2.25	0.99	1.41	0.96	1.67	0.96
76	2.40	0.99	2.80	0.99	2.32	0.99	1.45	0.97	1.72	0.97
77	2.46	0.99	2.88	0.99	2.38	0.99	1.49	0.97	1.77	0.97

Table A–6. Personality Inventory for DSM-5—Self-Report Form normative tables: trait scales *(continued)*

T	Anhedonia		Anxiousness		Attention seeking		Callousness		Deceitfulness	
	Raw	Percentile	Raw	Percentile	Raw	Percentile	Raw	Percentile	Raw	Percentile
78	2.52	0.99	2.95	1.00	2.44	0.99	1.54	0.97	1.82	0.98
79	2.58	0.99	3.02	1.00	2.50	0.99	1.58	0.97	1.87	0.98
80	2.64	1.00	3.09	1.00	2.57	0.99	1.62	0.97	1.92	0.98
81	2.70	1.00	3.16	1.00	2.63	1.00	1.66	0.98	1.96	0.98
82	2.76	1.00	3.24	1.00	2.69	1.00	1.71	0.98	2.01	0.99
83	2.82	1.00	3.31	1.00	2.75	1.00	1.75	0.98	2.06	0.99
84	2.88	1.00	3.38	1.00	2.82	1.00	1.79	0.98	2.11	0.99
85	2.94	1.00	3.45	1.00	2.88	1.00	1.83	0.98	2.16	0.99
86	3.00	1.00	3.53	1.00	2.94	1.00	1.88	0.98	2.21	0.99
87	3.06	1.00	3.60	1.00	3.01	1.00	1.92	0.98	2.26	0.99
88	3.12	1.00	3.67	1.00	3.07	1.00	1.96	0.99	2.31	0.99
89	3.18	1.00	3.74	1.00	3.13	1.00	2.00	0.99	2.36	0.99
90	3.24	1.00	3.81	1.00	3.19	1.00	2.05	0.99	2.41	0.99
91	3.30	1.00	3.89	1.00	3.26	1.00	2.09	1.00	2.45	0.99
92	3.36	1.00	3.96	1.00	3.32	1.00	2.13	1.00	2.50	0.99
93	3.42	1.00	4.00	1.00	3.38	1.00	2.17	1.00	2.55	0.99

Table A–6. Personality Inventory for DSM-5—Self-Report Form normative tables: trait scales (continued)

T	Anhedonia		Anxiousness		Attention seeking		Callousness		Deceitfulness	
	Raw	Percentile	Raw	Percentile	Raw	Percentile	Raw	Percentile	Raw	Percentile
94	3.48	1.00	4.00	1.00	3.45	1.00	2.22	1.00	2.60	1.00
95	3.54	1.00	4.00	1.00	3.51	1.00	2.26	1.00	2.65	1.00
96	3.60	1.00	4.00	1.00	3.57	1.00	2.30	1.00	2.70	1.00
97	3.66	1.00	4.00	1.00	3.63	1.00	2.34	1.00	2.75	1.00
98	3.72	1.00	4.00	1.00	3.70	1.00	2.39	1.00	2.80	1.00
99	3.78	1.00	4.00	1.00	3.76	1.00	2.43	1.00	2.85	1.00
100	3.84	1.00	4.00	1.00	3.82	1.00	2.47	1.00	2.89	1.00

T	Depressivity		Distractibility		Eccentricity		Emotional lability		Grandiosity	
	Raw	Percentile	Raw	Percentile	Raw	Percentile	Raw	Percentile	Raw	Percentile
30	0.00	0.00	0.00	0.00	0.00	0.00	0.00	0.00	0.00	0.00
31	0.00	0.00	0.00	0.00	0.00	0.00	0.00	0.00	0.00	0.00
32	0.00	0.00	0.00	0.00	0.00	0.00	0.00	0.00	0.00	0.00
33	0.00	0.00	0.00	0.00	0.00	0.00	0.00	0.00	0.00	0.00
34	0.00	0.00	0.00	0.00	0.00	0.00	0.00	0.00	0.00	0.00
35	0.00	0.00	0.00	0.00	0.00	0.00	0.00	0.00	0.00	0.00

Table A–6. Personality Inventory for DSM-5—Self-Report Form normative tables: trait scales *(continued)*

T	Depressivity		Distractibility		Eccentricity		Emotional lability		Grandiosity	
	Raw	Percentile	Raw	Percentile	Raw	Percentile	Raw	Percentile	Raw	Percentile
36	0.00	0.00	0.00	0.00	0.00	0.00	0.00	0.00	0.00	0.00
37	0.00	0.00	0.00	0.00	0.00	0.00	0.00	0.00	0.00	0.00
38	0.00	0.00	0.00	0.00	0.00	0.00	0.00	0.00	0.04	0.13
39	0.00	0.00	0.02	0.13	0.00	0.00	0.04	0.13	0.10	0.13
40	0.00	0.00	0.09	0.13	0.00	0.00	0.10	0.13	0.15	0.13
41	0.00	0.00	0.15	0.21	0.00	0.21	0.17	0.23	0.21	0.23
42	0.00	0.00	0.22	0.21	0.07	0.21	0.24	0.23	0.27	0.23
43	0.05	0.25	0.29	0.30	0.15	0.29	0.31	0.33	0.32	0.23
44	0.11	0.36	0.35	0.38	0.22	0.37	0.38	0.34	0.38	0.35
45	0.16	0.47	0.42	0.38	0.30	0.43	0.45	0.42	0.44	0.35
46	0.22	0.52	0.48	0.45	0.37	0.48	0.52	0.43	0.49	0.35
47	0.27	0.53	0.55	0.45	0.45	0.53	0.59	0.50	0.55	0.47
48	0.33	0.59	0.62	0.51	0.52	0.56	0.66	0.50	0.61	0.47
49	0.38	0.62	0.68	0.56	0.59	0.59	0.73	0.59	0.66	0.47
50	0.44	0.68	0.75	0.56	0.67	0.62	0.80	0.59	0.72	0.58
51	0.49	0.68	0.82	0.61	0.74	0.64	0.87	0.64	0.77	0.58

Table A–6. Personality Inventory for DSM-5—Self-Report Form normative tables: trait scales (*continued*)

T	Depressivity		Distractibility		Eccentricity		Emotional lability		Grandiosity	
	Raw	Percentile	Raw	Percentile	Raw	Percentile	Raw	Percentile	Raw	Percentile
52	0.55	0.71	0.88	0.62	0.82	0.67	0.94	0.64	0.83	0.59
53	0.60	0.73	0.95	0.66	0.89	0.71	1.01	0.69	0.89	0.68
54	0.66	0.77	1.01	0.72	0.96	0.72	1.08	0.69	0.94	0.68
55	0.71	0.77	1.08	0.72	1.04	0.75	1.15	0.76	1.00	0.68
56	0.76	0.79	1.15	0.77	1.11	0.76	1.22	0.76	1.06	0.76
57	0.82	0.81	1.21	0.77	1.19	0.79	1.29	0.79	1.11	0.76
58	0.87	0.83	1.28	0.80	1.26	0.81	1.36	0.79	1.17	0.83
59	0.93	0.85	1.35	0.83	1.33	0.82	1.43	0.83	1.22	0.83
60	0.98	0.85	1.41	0.83	1.41	0.83	1.50	0.83	1.28	0.83
61	1.04	0.86	1.48	0.85	1.48	0.85	1.57	0.83	1.34	0.87
62	1.09	0.88	1.54	0.85	1.56	0.86	1.64	0.86	1.39	0.87
63	1.15	0.89	1.61	0.88	1.63	0.87	1.71	0.86	1.45	0.88
64	1.20	0.89	1.68	0.91	1.71	0.89	1.78	0.89	1.51	0.91
65	1.26	0.90	1.74	0.91	1.78	0.91	1.85	0.89	1.56	0.91
66	1.31	0.92	1.81	0.93	1.85	0.91	1.92	0.92	1.62	0.91
67	1.37	0.93	1.88	0.94	1.93	0.93	1.99	0.92	1.67	0.94

Table A–6. Personality Inventory for DSM-5—Self-Report Form normative tables: trait scales *(continued)*

T	Depressivity		Distractibility		Eccentricity		Emotional lability		Grandiosity	
	Raw	Percentile	Raw	Percentile	Raw	Percentile	Raw	Percentile	Raw	Percentile
68	1.42	0.93	1.94	0.95	2.00	0.93	2.06	0.94	1.73	0.94
69	1.48	0.94	2.01	0.96	2.08	0.93	2.13	0.94	1.79	0.95
70	1.53	0.94	2.08	0.96	2.15	0.94	2.20	0.95	1.84	0.97
71	1.58	0.94	2.14	0.96	2.22	0.95	2.27	0.95	1.90	0.97
72	1.64	0.94	2.21	0.96	2.30	0.95	2.34	0.96	1.96	0.97
73	1.69	0.95	2.27	0.97	2.37	0.95	2.41	0.96	2.01	0.98
74	1.75	0.96	2.34	0.97	2.45	0.96	2.48	0.97	2.07	0.98
75	1.80	0.96	2.41	0.97	2.52	0.96	2.55	0.97	2.12	0.98
76	1.86	0.97	2.47	0.97	2.59	0.96	2.62	0.98	2.18	0.99
77	1.91	0.97	2.54	0.97	2.67	0.98	2.69	0.98	2.24	0.99
78	1.97	0.97	2.61	0.98	2.74	0.98	2.76	0.99	2.29	0.99
79	2.02	0.98	2.67	0.98	2.82	0.98	2.83	0.99	2.35	0.99
80	2.08	0.98	2.74	0.98	2.89	0.98	2.90	1.00	2.41	0.99
81	2.13	0.98	2.80	0.99	2.96	0.99	2.97	1.00	2.46	0.99
82	2.19	0.98	2.87	0.99	3.04	1.00	3.04	1.00	2.52	1.00
83	2.24	0.99	2.94	0.99	3.11	1.00	3.10	1.00	2.58	1.00

Table A–6. Personality Inventory for DSM-5—Self-Report Form normative tables: trait scales (continued)

T	Depressivity Raw	Percentile	Distractibility Raw	Percentile	Eccentricity Raw	Percentile	Emotional lability Raw	Percentile	Grandiosity Raw	Percentile
84	2.30	0.99	3.00	1.00	3.19	1.00	3.17	1.00	2.63	1.00
85	2.35	0.99	3.07	1.00	3.26	1.00	3.24	1.00	2.69	1.00
86	2.40	0.99	3.14	1.00	3.34	1.00	3.31	1.00	2.74	1.00
87	2.46	0.99	3.20	1.00	3.41	1.00	3.38	1.00	2.80	1.00
88	2.51	1.00	3.27	1.00	3.48	1.00	3.45	1.00	2.86	1.00
89	2.57	1.00	3.33	1.00	3.56	1.00	3.52	1.00	2.91	1.00
90	2.62	1.00	3.40	1.00	3.63	1.00	3.59	1.00	2.97	1.00
91	2.68	1.00	3.47	1.00	3.71	1.00	3.66	1.00	3.03	1.00
92	2.73	1.00	3.53	1.00	3.78	1.00	3.73	1.00	3.08	1.00
93	2.79	1.00	3.60	1.00	3.85	1.00	3.80	1.00	3.14	1.00
94	2.84	1.00	3.67	1.00	3.93	1.00	3.87	1.00	3.19	1.00
95	2.90	1.00	3.73	1.00	4.00	1.00	3.94	1.00	3.25	1.00
96	2.95	1.00	3.80	1.00	4.00	1.00	4.00	1.00	3.31	1.00
97	3.01	1.00	3.86	1.00	4.00	1.00	4.00	1.00	3.36	1.00
98	3.06	1.00	3.93	1.00	4.00	1.00	4.00	1.00	3.42	1.00
99	3.12	1.00	4.00	1.00	4.00	1.00	4.00	1.00	3.48	1.00
100	3.17	1.00	4.00	1.00	4.00	1.00	4.00	1.00	3.53	1.00

Table A–6. Personality Inventory for DSM-5—Self-Report Form normative tables: trait scales *(continued)*

T	Hostility		Impulsivity		Intimacy avoidance		Irresponsibility		Manipulativeness	
	Raw	Percentile	Raw	Percentile	Raw	Percentile	Raw	Percentile	Raw	Percentile
30	0.00	0.00	0.00	0.00	0.00	0.00	0.00	0.00	0.00	0.00
31	0.00	0.00	0.00	0.00	0.00	0.00	0.00	0.00	0.00	0.00
32	0.00	0.00	0.00	0.00	0.00	0.00	0.00	0.00	0.00	0.00
33	0.00	0.00	0.00	0.00	0.00	0.00	0.00	0.00	0.00	0.00
34	0.00	0.00	0.00	0.00	0.00	0.00	0.00	0.00	0.00	0.00
35	0.00	0.00	0.00	0.00	0.00	0.00	0.00	0.00	0.00	0.00
36	0.00	0.00	0.00	0.00	0.00	0.00	0.00	0.00	0.00	0.00
37	0.00	0.06	0.00	0.00	0.00	0.00	0.00	0.00	0.00	0.00
38	0.06	0.06	0.00	0.00	0.00	0.00	0.00	0.00	0.00	0.00
39	0.13	0.11	0.00	0.17	0.00	0.00	0.00	0.00	0.02	0.20
40	0.19	0.11	0.06	0.17	0.00	0.00	0.00	0.00	0.08	0.20
41	0.25	0.20	0.12	0.17	0.00	0.00	0.00	0.00	0.14	0.20
42	0.32	0.26	0.18	0.29	0.01	0.39	0.00	0.00	0.21	0.31
43	0.38	0.27	0.24	0.30	0.07	0.39	0.03	0.39	0.27	0.32
44	0.44	0.33	0.30	0.30	0.14	0.39	0.07	0.39	0.33	0.32
45	0.51	0.41	0.36	0.44	0.20	0.52	0.11	0.39	0.40	0.32

Table A–6. Personality Inventory for DSM-5—Self-Report Form normative tables: trait scales *(continued)*

T	Hostility Raw	Hostility Percentile	Impulsivity Raw	Impulsivity Percentile	Intimacy avoidance Raw	Intimacy avoidance Percentile	Irresponsibility Raw	Irresponsibility Percentile	Manipulativeness Raw	Manipulativeness Percentile
46	0.57	0.41	0.42	0.44	0.27	0.52	0.16	0.54	0.46	0.44
47	0.63	0.48	0.48	0.44	0.33	0.52	0.20	0.55	0.53	0.45
48	0.70	0.48	0.54	0.54	0.39	0.52	0.24	0.55	0.59	0.45
49	0.76	0.53	0.61	0.55	0.46	0.61	0.28	0.55	0.65	0.57
50	0.82	0.59	0.67	0.55	0.52	0.61	0.33	0.65	0.72	0.57
51	0.89	0.59	0.73	0.63	0.59	0.61	0.37	0.66	0.78	0.57
52	0.95	0.64	0.79	0.64	0.65	0.69	0.41	0.66	0.84	0.67
53	1.01	0.70	0.85	0.72	0.72	0.69	0.46	0.75	0.91	0.67
54	1.07	0.70	0.91	0.72	0.78	0.70	0.50	0.75	0.97	0.67
55	1.14	0.74	0.97	0.72	0.84	0.77	0.54	0.75	1.03	0.74
56	1.20	0.77	1.03	0.78	0.91	0.77	0.58	0.81	1.10	0.74
57	1.26	0.77	1.09	0.78	0.97	0.77	0.63	0.81	1.16	0.74
58	1.33	0.80	1.15	0.78	1.04	0.83	0.67	0.81	1.22	0.82
59	1.39	0.80	1.21	0.84	1.10	0.83	0.71	0.81	1.29	0.82
60	1.45	0.84	1.27	0.84	1.17	0.83	0.75	0.86	1.35	0.82
61	1.52	0.87	1.33	0.84	1.23	0.87	0.80	0.86	1.41	0.87

Table A–6. Personality Inventory for DSM-5—Self-Report Form normative tables: trait scales *(continued)*

T	Hostility		Impulsivity		Intimacy avoidance		Irresponsibility		Manipulativeness	
	Raw	Percentile	Raw	Percentile	Raw	Percentile	Raw	Percentile	Raw	Percentile
62	1.58	0.88	1.39	0.87	1.30	0.87	0.84	0.87	1.48	0.87
63	1.64	0.90	1.45	0.87	1.36	0.87	0.88	0.90	1.54	0.87
64	1.71	0.91	1.51	0.90	1.42	0.90	0.92	0.90	1.60	0.91
65	1.77	0.91	1.57	0.90	1.49	0.90	0.97	0.90	1.67	0.91
66	1.83	0.92	1.63	0.90	1.55	0.90	1.01	0.94	1.73	0.91
67	1.90	0.92	1.69	0.93	1.62	0.92	1.05	0.94	1.79	0.92
68	1.96	0.94	1.75	0.93	1.68	0.92	1.09	0.94	1.86	0.96
69	2.02	0.95	1.81	0.93	1.75	0.92	1.14	0.94	1.92	0.96
70	2.08	0.95	1.87	0.95	1.81	0.95	1.18	0.95	1.99	0.96
71	2.15	0.95	1.93	0.95	1.87	0.95	1.22	0.95	2.05	0.98
72	2.21	0.96	1.99	0.95	1.94	0.95	1.26	0.95	2.11	0.98
73	2.27	0.96	2.05	0.97	2.00	0.96	1.31	0.96	2.18	0.98
74	2.34	0.97	2.11	0.97	2.07	0.96	1.35	0.97	2.24	0.98
75	2.40	0.98	2.17	0.98	2.13	0.96	1.39	0.97	2.30	0.98
76	2.46	0.98	2.23	0.98	2.20	0.96	1.43	0.98	2.37	0.98
77	2.53	0.98	2.29	0.98	2.26	0.98	1.48	0.98	2.43	0.99

Table A–6. Personality Inventory for DSM-5—Self-Report Form normative tables: trait scales *(continued)*

T	Hostility Raw	Hostility Percentile	Impulsivity Raw	Impulsivity Percentile	Intimacy avoidance Raw	Intimacy avoidance Percentile	Irresponsibility Raw	Irresponsibility Percentile	Manipulativeness Raw	Manipulativeness Percentile
78	2.59	0.98	2.35	0.99	2.32	0.98	1.52	0.98	2.49	0.99
79	2.65	0.99	2.41	0.99	2.39	0.98	1.56	0.98	2.56	0.99
80	2.72	0.99	2.47	0.99	2.45	0.99	1.61	0.98	2.62	0.99
81	2.78	0.99	2.53	1.00	2.52	0.99	1.65	0.98	2.68	0.99
82	2.84	0.99	2.59	1.00	2.58	0.99	1.69	0.98	2.75	0.99
83	2.91	0.99	2.65	1.00	2.65	1.00	1.73	0.98	2.81	0.99
84	2.97	0.99	2.71	1.00	2.71	1.00	1.78	0.98	2.87	0.99
85	3.03	1.00	2.77	1.00	2.77	1.00	1.82	0.98	2.94	0.99
86	3.09	1.00	2.83	1.00	2.84	1.00	1.86	0.99	3.00	1.00
87	3.16	1.00	2.89	1.00	2.90	1.00	1.90	0.99	3.06	1.00
88	3.22	1.00	2.96	1.00	2.97	1.00	1.95	0.99	3.13	1.00
89	3.28	1.00	3.02	1.00	3.03	1.00	1.99	0.99	3.19	1.00
90	3.35	1.00	3.08	1.00	3.10	1.00	2.03	0.99	3.25	1.00
91	3.41	1.00	3.14	1.00	3.16	1.00	2.07	0.99	3.32	1.00
92	3.47	1.00	3.20	1.00	3.22	1.00	2.12	0.99	3.38	1.00
93	3.54	1.00	3.26	1.00	3.29	1.00	2.16	1.00	3.45	1.00

Table A–6. Personality Inventory for DSM-5—Self-Report Form normative tables: trait scales *(continued)*

T	Hostility		Impulsivity		Intimacy avoidance		Irresponsibility		Manipulativeness	
	Raw	Percentile	Raw	Percentile	Raw	Percentile	Raw	Percentile	Raw	Percentile
94	3.60	1.00	3.32	1.00	3.35	1.00	2.20	1.00	3.51	1.00
95	3.66	1.00	3.38	1.00	3.42	1.00	2.24	1.00	3.57	1.00
96	3.73	1.00	3.44	1.00	3.48	1.00	2.29	1.00	3.64	1.00
97	3.79	1.00	3.50	1.00	3.55	1.00	2.33	1.00	3.70	1.00
98	3.85	1.00	3.56	1.00	3.61	1.00	2.37	1.00	3.76	1.00
99	3.92	1.00	3.62	1.00	3.67	1.00	2.41	1.00	3.83	1.00
100	3.98	1.00	3.68	1.00	3.74	1.00	2.46	1.00	3.89	1.00

T	Perceptual dysregulation		Perseveration		Restricted affectivity		Rigid perfectionism		Risk taking	
	Raw	Percentile	Raw	Percentile	Raw	Percentile	Raw	Percentile	Raw	Percentile
30	0.00	0.00	0.00	0.00	0.00	0.00	0.00	0.00	0.00	0.00
31	0.00	0.00	0.00	0.00	0.00	0.00	0.00	0.00	0.03	0.01
32	0.00	0.00	0.00	0.00	0.00	0.00	0.00	0.00	0.08	0.02
33	0.00	0.00	0.00	0.00	0.00	0.00	0.00	0.00	0.13	0.02
34	0.00	0.00	0.00	0.00	0.00	0.00	0.00	0.00	0.18	0.04
35	0.00	0.00	0.00	0.00	0.02	0.07	0.00	0.00	0.23	0.05

Table A–6. Personality Inventory for DSM-5—Self-Report Form normative tables: trait scales (continued)

T	Perceptual dysregulation Raw	Percentile	Perseveration Raw	Percentile	Restricted affectivity Raw	Percentile	Rigid perfectionism Raw	Percentile	Risk taking Raw	Percentile
36	0.00	0.00	0.00	0.00	0.08	0.07	0.01	0.05	0.29	0.08
37	0.00	0.00	0.00	0.00	0.14	0.07	0.08	0.05	0.34	0.08
38	0.00	0.00	0.00	0.00	0.20	0.13	0.15	0.10	0.39	0.11
39	0.00	0.00	0.05	0.14	0.25	0.13	0.22	0.16	0.44	0.13
40	0.00	0.00	0.11	0.22	0.31	0.20	0.28	0.16	0.49	0.13
41	0.00	0.00	0.17	0.23	0.37	0.20	0.35	0.22	0.54	0.18
42	0.00	0.27	0.23	0.32	0.43	0.20	0.42	0.28	0.59	0.22
43	0.05	0.27	0.29	0.32	0.48	0.27	0.49	0.28	0.64	0.27
44	0.09	0.42	0.35	0.38	0.54	0.27	0.56	0.34	0.70	0.28
45	0.13	0.43	0.41	0.39	0.60	0.37	0.63	0.39	0.75	0.34
46	0.18	0.53	0.47	0.44	0.66	0.37	0.70	0.40	0.80	0.40
47	0.22	0.53	0.53	0.45	0.72	0.46	0.76	0.45	0.85	0.40
48	0.26	0.60	0.59	0.50	0.77	0.46	0.83	0.48	0.90	0.45
49	0.30	0.61	0.65	0.50	0.83	0.46	0.90	0.53	0.95	0.51
50	0.35	0.68	0.71	0.56	0.89	0.58	0.97	0.53	1.00	0.57
51	0.39	0.68	0.77	0.56	0.95	0.58	1.04	0.59	1.05	0.57

Table A–6. Personality Inventory for DSM-5—Self-Report Form normative tables: trait scales *(continued)*

T	Perceptual dysregulation		Perseveration		Restricted affectivity		Rigid perfectionism		Risk taking	
	Raw	Percentile	Raw	Percentile	Raw	Percentile	Raw	Percentile	Raw	Percentile
52	0.43	0.73	0.83	0.61	1.00	0.66	1.11	0.64	1.10	0.63
53	0.48	0.73	0.89	0.66	1.06	0.66	1.18	0.64	1.16	0.67
54	0.52	0.77	0.95	0.66	1.12	0.66	1.24	0.68	1.21	0.67
55	0.56	0.77	1.01	0.71	1.18	0.72	1.31	0.71	1.26	0.72
56	0.60	0.80	1.07	0.71	1.24	0.72	1.38	0.71	1.31	0.74
57	0.65	0.80	1.13	0.77	1.29	0.78	1.45	0.75	1.36	0.79
58	0.69	0.83	1.19	0.77	1.35	0.78	1.52	0.78	1.41	0.79
59	0.73	0.83	1.25	0.82	1.41	0.78	1.59	0.78	1.46	0.82
60	0.77	0.85	1.31	0.82	1.47	0.84	1.65	0.81	1.51	0.85
61	0.82	0.85	1.37	0.86	1.52	0.84	1.72	0.85	1.56	0.85
62	0.86	0.87	1.43	0.86	1.58	0.89	1.79	0.85	1.62	0.87
63	0.90	0.88	1.49	0.89	1.64	0.89	1.86	0.87	1.67	0.90
64	0.95	0.89	1.55	0.89	1.70	0.89	1.93	0.91	1.72	0.92
65	0.99	0.89	1.61	0.91	1.75	0.93	2.00	0.91	1.77	0.92
66	1.03	0.91	1.67	0.93	1.81	0.93	2.07	0.92	1.82	0.94
67	1.07	0.91	1.73	0.93	1.87	0.96	2.13	0.94	1.87	0.95

Table A–6. Personality Inventory for DSM-5—Self-Report Form normative tables: trait scales (continued)

T	Perceptual dysregulation		Perseveration		Restricted affectivity		Rigid perfectionism		Risk taking	
	Raw	Percentile	Raw	Percentile	Raw	Percentile	Raw	Percentile	Raw	Percentile
68	1.12	0.93	1.79	0.95	1.93	0.96	2.20	0.96	1.92	0.95
69	1.16	0.93	1.85	0.95	1.99	0.96	2.27	0.96	1.97	0.96
70	1.20	0.94	1.91	0.96	2.04	0.97	2.34	0.97	2.03	0.97
71	1.25	0.94	1.97	0.96	2.10	0.97	2.41	0.98	2.08	0.97
72	1.29	0.96	2.03	0.98	2.16	0.98	2.48	0.98	2.13	0.97
73	1.33	0.96	2.09	0.98	2.22	0.98	2.54	0.98	2.18	0.98
74	1.37	0.96	2.15	0.98	2.27	0.98	2.61	0.99	2.23	0.99
75	1.42	0.97	2.21	0.98	2.33	0.99	2.68	0.99	2.28	0.99
76	1.46	0.97	2.27	0.99	2.39	0.99	2.75	0.99	2.33	0.99
77	1.50	0.97	2.33	0.99	2.45	0.99	2.82	1.00	2.38	0.99
78	1.55	0.97	2.39	0.99	2.51	0.99	2.89	1.00	2.43	0.99
79	1.59	0.98	2.45	1.00	2.56	0.99	2.96	1.00	2.49	0.99
80	1.63	0.98	2.51	1.00	2.62	1.00	3.02	1.00	2.54	0.99
81	1.67	0.98	2.57	1.00	2.68	1.00	3.09	1.00	2.59	0.99
82	1.72	0.98	2.63	1.00	2.74	1.00	3.16	1.00	2.64	0.99
83	1.76	0.99	2.69	1.00	2.79	1.00	3.23	1.00	2.69	1.00
84	1.80	0.99	2.75	1.00	2.85	1.00	3.30	1.00	2.74	1.00

Table A–6. Personality Inventory for DSM-5—Self-Report Form normative tables: trait scales *(continued)*

T	Perceptual dysregulation Raw	Percentile	Perseveration Raw	Percentile	Restricted affectivity Raw	Percentile	Rigid perfectionism Raw	Percentile	Risk taking Raw	Percentile
85	1.84	0.99	2.81	1.00	2.91	1.00	3.37	1.00	2.79	1.00
86	1.89	0.99	2.87	1.00	2.97	1.00	3.44	1.00	2.84	1.00
87	1.93	1.00	2.93	1.00	3.02	1.00	3.50	1.00	2.89	1.00
88	1.97	1.00	2.99	1.00	3.08	1.00	3.57	1.00	2.95	1.00
89	2.02	1.00	3.05	1.00	3.14	1.00	3.64	1.00	3.00	1.00
90	2.06	1.00	3.11	1.00	3.20	1.00	3.71	1.00	3.05	1.00
91	2.10	1.00	3.17	1.00	3.26	1.00	3.78	1.00	3.10	1.00
92	2.14	1.00	3.23	1.00	3.31	1.00	3.85	1.00	3.15	1.00
93	2.19	1.00	3.29	1.00	3.37	1.00	3.91	1.00	3.20	1.00
94	2.23	1.00	3.35	1.00	3.43	1.00	3.98	1.00	3.25	1.00
95	2.27	1.00	3.41	1.00	3.49	1.00	4.00	1.00	3.30	1.00
96	2.32	1.00	3.47	1.00	3.54	1.00	4.00	1.00	3.36	1.00
97	2.36	1.00	3.53	1.00	3.60	1.00	4.00	1.00	3.41	1.00
98	2.40	1.00	3.59	1.00	3.66	1.00	4.00	1.00	3.46	1.00
99	2.44	1.00	3.65	1.00	3.72	1.00	4.00	1.00	3.51	1.00
100	2.49	1.00	3.70	1.00	3.78	1.00	4.00	1.00	3.56	1.00

Table A–6. Personality Inventory for DSM-5 — Self-Report Form normative tables: trait scales *(continued)*

T	Separation insecurity		Submissiveness		Suspiciousness		Unusual beliefs and experiences		Withdrawal	
	Raw	Percentile	Raw	Percentile	Raw	Percentile	Raw	Percentile	Raw	Percentile
30	0.00	0.00	0.00	0.00	0.00	0.00	0.00	0.00	0.00	0.00
31	0.00	0.00	0.00	0.00	0.00	0.00	0.00	0.00	0.00	0.00
32	0.00	0.00	0.00	0.00	0.00	0.00	0.00	0.00	0.00	0.00
33	0.00	0.00	0.00	0.00	0.00	0.00	0.00	0.00	0.00	0.00
34	0.00	0.00	0.01	0.09	0.00	0.00	0.00	0.00	0.00	0.00
35	0.00	0.00	0.08	0.09	0.00	0.00	0.00	0.00	0.00	0.00
36	0.00	0.00	0.15	0.09	0.00	0.09	0.00	0.00	0.00	0.00
37	0.00	0.00	0.22	0.09	0.06	0.09	0.00	0.00	0.02	0.07
38	0.00	0.00	0.29	0.18	0.12	0.09	0.00	0.00	0.09	0.07
39	0.00	0.17	0.35	0.19	0.18	0.18	0.00	0.00	0.16	0.14
40	0.07	0.17	0.42	0.19	0.24	0.18	0.00	0.00	0.23	0.20
41	0.13	0.17	0.49	0.19	0.30	0.18	0.00	0.00	0.30	0.27
42	0.19	0.27	0.56	0.28	0.35	0.27	0.05	0.28	0.37	0.28
43	0.26	0.27	0.63	0.28	0.41	0.28	0.11	0.28	0.44	0.32
44	0.32	0.39	0.70	0.28	0.47	0.28	0.16	0.40	0.51	0.36
45	0.38	0.39	0.76	0.39	0.53	0.40	0.22	0.40	0.59	0.36

Table A–6. Personality Inventory for DSM-5—Self-Report Form normative tables: trait scales *(continued)*

T	Separation insecurity		Submissiveness		Suspiciousness		Unusual beliefs and experiences		Withdrawal	
	Raw	Percentile	Raw	Percentile	Raw	Percentile	Raw	Percentile	Raw	Percentile
46	0.45	0.48	0.83	0.39	0.59	0.40	0.27	0.51	0.66	0.42
47	0.51	0.48	0.90	0.39	0.65	0.41	0.32	0.51	0.73	0.47
48	0.57	0.55	0.97	0.39	0.70	0.50	0.38	0.59	0.80	0.47
49	0.64	0.56	1.04	0.52	0.76	0.50	0.43	0.59	0.87	0.50
50	0.70	0.56	1.11	0.52	0.82	0.50	0.49	0.59	0.94	0.55
51	0.76	0.62	1.17	0.52	0.88	0.61	0.54	0.66	1.01	0.60
52	0.83	0.62	1.24	0.52	0.94	0.61	0.60	0.67	1.08	0.60
53	0.89	0.69	1.31	0.62	1.00	0.61	0.65	0.72	1.16	0.64
54	0.95	0.69	1.38	0.63	1.05	0.70	0.71	0.72	1.23	0.68
55	1.02	0.74	1.45	0.63	1.11	0.70	0.76	0.77	1.30	0.68
56	1.08	0.74	1.52	0.73	1.17	0.77	0.82	0.77	1.37	0.70
57	1.15	0.79	1.58	0.73	1.23	0.78	0.87	0.77	1.44	0.75
58	1.21	0.79	1.65	0.73	1.29	0.78	0.92	0.80	1.51	0.78
59	1.27	0.79	1.72	0.73	1.35	0.83	0.98	0.80	1.58	0.78
60	1.34	0.85	1.79	0.85	1.40	0.84	1.03	0.84	1.65	0.82
61	1.40	0.85	1.86	0.85	1.46	0.84	1.09	0.84	1.73	0.86

Table A–6. Personality Inventory for DSM-5—Self-Report Form normative tables: trait scales *(continued)*

T	Separation insecurity		Submissiveness		Suspiciousness		Unusual beliefs and experiences		Withdrawal	
	Raw	Percentile	Raw	Percentile	Raw	Percentile	Raw	Percentile	Raw	Percentile
62	1.46	0.87	1.93	0.85	1.52	0.88	1.14	0.87	1.80	0.86
63	1.53	0.87	2.00	0.85	1.58	0.88	1.20	0.87	1.87	0.88
64	1.59	0.90	2.06	0.94	1.64	0.89	1.25	0.91	1.94	0.91
65	1.65	0.90	2.13	0.94	1.70	0.93	1.31	0.91	2.01	0.92
66	1.72	0.92	2.20	0.94	1.75	0.93	1.36	0.91	2.08	0.92
67	1.78	0.92	2.27	0.98	1.81	0.93	1.42	0.93	2.15	0.93
68	1.84	0.92	2.34	0.98	1.87	0.95	1.47	0.93	2.22	0.95
69	1.91	0.94	2.41	0.98	1.93	0.95	1.52	0.95	2.30	0.95
70	1.97	0.94	2.47	0.98	1.99	0.95	1.58	0.95	2.37	0.96
71	2.03	0.96	2.54	0.99	2.04	0.97	1.63	0.95	2.44	0.97
72	2.10	0.96	2.61	0.99	2.10	0.97	1.69	0.95	2.51	0.98
73	2.16	0.97	2.68	0.99	2.16	0.97	1.74	0.95	2.58	0.98
74	2.22	0.97	2.75	0.99	2.22	0.98	1.80	0.97	2.65	0.98
75	2.29	0.98	2.82	1.00	2.28	0.98	1.85	0.97	2.72	0.99
76	2.35	0.99	2.88	1.00	2.34	0.99	1.91	0.98	2.79	0.99
77	2.42	0.99	2.95	1.00	2.39	0.99	1.96	0.98	2.87	0.99

Table A–6. Personality Inventory for DSM-5—Self-Report Form normative tables: trait scales *(continued)*

T	Separation insecurity Raw	Percentile	Submissiveness Raw	Percentile	Suspiciousness Raw	Percentile	Unusual beliefs and experiences Raw	Percentile	Withdrawal Raw	Percentile
78	2.48	0.99	3.02	1.00	2.45	0.99	2.02	0.99	2.94	0.99
79	2.54	0.99	3.09	1.00	2.51	0.99	2.07	0.99	3.01	1.00
80	2.61	1.00	3.16	1.00	2.57	0.99	2.12	0.99	3.08	1.00
81	2.67	1.00	3.23	1.00	2.63	1.00	2.18	0.99	3.15	1.00
82	2.73	1.00	3.29	1.00	2.69	1.00	2.23	0.99	3.22	1.00
83	2.80	1.00	3.36	1.00	2.74	1.00	2.29	0.99	3.29	1.00
84	2.86	1.00	3.43	1.00	2.80	1.00	2.34	0.99	3.36	1.00
85	2.92	1.00	3.50	1.00	2.86	1.00	2.40	0.99	3.44	1.00
86	2.99	1.00	3.57	1.00	2.92	1.00	2.45	0.99	3.51	1.00
87	3.05	1.00	3.64	1.00	2.98	1.00	2.51	1.00	3.58	1.00
88	3.11	1.00	3.70	1.00	3.04	1.00	2.56	1.00	3.65	1.00
89	3.18	1.00	3.77	1.00	3.09	1.00	2.62	1.00	3.72	1.00
90	3.24	1.00	3.84	1.00	3.15	1.00	2.67	1.00	3.79	1.00
91	3.30	1.00	3.91	1.00	3.21	1.00	2.72	1.00	3.86	1.00
92	3.37	1.00	3.98	1.00	3.27	1.00	2.78	1.00	3.93	1.00
93	3.43	1.00	4.00	1.00	3.33	1.00	2.83	1.00	4.00	1.00

Table A–6. Personality Inventory for DSM-5—Self-Report Form normative tables: trait scales *(continued)*

T	Separation insecurity		Submissiveness		Suspiciousness		Unusual beliefs and experiences		Withdrawal	
	Raw	Percentile	Raw	Percentile	Raw	Percentile	Raw	Percentile	Raw	Percentile
94	3.50	1.00	4.00	1.00	3.39	1.00	2.89	1.00	4.00	1.00
95	3.56	1.00	4.00	1.00	3.44	1.00	2.94	1.00	4.00	1.00
96	3.62	1.00	4.00	1.00	3.50	1.00	3.00	1.00	4.00	1.00
97	3.69	1.00	4.00	1.00	3.56	1.00	3.05	1.00	4.00	1.00
98	3.75	1.00	4.00	1.00	3.62	1.00	3.11	1.00	4.00	1.00
99	3.81	1.00	4.00	1.00	3.68	1.00	3.16	1.00	4.00	1.00
100	3.88	1.00	4.00	1.00	3.74	1.00	3.22	1.00	4.00	1.00

Table A–7. Personality Inventory for DSM-5—Self-Report Form (100 item) normative tables: domain scales

T	Negative affect		Detachment		Antagonism		Disinhibition		Psychoticism	
	Raw	Percentile	Raw	Percentile	Raw	Percentile	Raw	Percentile	Raw	Percentile
30	0.00	0.00	0.00	0.00	0.00	0.00	0.00	0.00	0.00	0.00
31	0.00	0.00	0.00	0.00	0.00	0.00	0.00	0.00	0.00	0.00
32	0.00	0.00	0.00	0.00	0.00	0.00	0.00	0.00	0.00	0.00
33	0.00	0.00	0.00	0.00	0.00	0.00	0.00	0.00	0.00	0.00
34	0.00	0.00	0.00	0.00	0.00	0.00	0.00	0.00	0.00	0.00
35	0.00	0.00	0.00	0.00	0.00	0.00	0.00	0.00	0.00	0.00
36	0.00	0.00	0.00	0.00	0.00	0.00	0.00	0.00	0.00	0.00
37	0.00	0.00	0.00	0.00	0.00	0.00	0.00	0.00	0.00	0.00
38	0.00	0.00	0.00	0.00	0.00	0.00	0.00	0.00	0.00	0.00
39	0.04	0.11	0.00	0.16	0.00	0.00	0.01	0.11	0.00	0.00
40	0.11	0.18	0.06	0.16	0.02	0.13	0.06	0.11	0.00	0.00
41	0.17	0.24	0.12	0.22	0.07	0.13	0.11	0.21	0.00	0.00
42	0.24	0.24	0.17	0.30	0.11	0.22	0.16	0.21	0.00	0.31
43	0.30	0.30	0.23	0.30	0.16	0.22	0.21	0.28	0.05	0.31
44	0.37	0.37	0.29	0.36	0.21	0.35	0.26	0.36	0.10	0.43

Table A–7. Personality Inventory for DSM-5—Self-Report Form (100 item) normative tables: domain scales *(continued)*

T	Negative affect		Detachment		Antagonism		Disinhibition		Psychoticism	
	Raw	Percentile	Raw	Percentile	Raw	Percentile	Raw	Percentile	Raw	Percentile
45	0.43	0.41	0.35	0.42	0.26	0.44	0.31	0.36	0.14	0.43
46	0.49	0.41	0.40	0.42	0.31	0.44	0.36	0.45	0.19	0.52
47	0.56	0.46	0.46	0.48	0.35	0.52	0.41	0.45	0.24	0.52
48	0.62	0.51	0.52	0.52	0.40	0.52	0.46	0.53	0.29	0.58
49	0.69	0.55	0.58	0.52	0.45	0.58	0.51	0.59	0.34	0.64
50	0.75	0.58	0.63	0.58	0.50	0.58	0.56	0.59	0.38	0.64
51	0.82	0.58	0.69	0.62	0.54	0.64	0.61	0.64	0.43	0.69
52	0.88	0.61	0.75	0.62	0.59	0.68	0.66	0.65	0.48	0.69
53	0.94	0.67	0.81	0.67	0.64	0.68	0.71	0.68	0.53	0.73
54	1.01	0.72	0.86	0.71	0.69	0.74	0.76	0.74	0.57	0.73
55	1.07	0.72	0.92	0.74	0.74	0.74	0.81	0.74	0.62	0.77
56	1.14	0.76	0.98	0.74	0.78	0.78	0.86	0.77	0.67	0.79
57	1.20	0.80	1.04	0.77	0.83	0.79	0.91	0.77	0.72	0.79
58	1.27	0.82	1.09	0.80	0.88	0.82	0.96	0.80	0.77	0.83
59	1.33	0.82	1.15	0.80	0.93	0.85	1.01	0.84	0.81	0.83

Table A–7. Personality Inventory for DSM-5—Self-Report Form (100 item) normative tables: domain scales *(continued)*

T	Negative affect		Detachment		Antagonism		Disinhibition		Psychoticism	
	Raw	Percentile	Raw	Percentile	Raw	Percentile	Raw	Percentile	Raw	Percentile
60	1.40	0.84	1.21	0.83	0.97	0.85	1.05	0.84	0.86	0.85
61	1.46	0.86	1.27	0.84	1.02	0.87	1.10	0.86	0.91	0.85
62	1.52	0.87	1.32	0.84	1.07	0.87	1.15	0.86	0.96	0.86
63	1.59	0.89	1.38	0.87	1.12	0.89	1.20	0.89	1.00	0.89
64	1.65	0.89	1.44	0.89	1.17	0.89	1.25	0.90	1.05	0.89
65	1.72	0.89	1.50	0.89	1.21	0.91	1.30	0.90	1.10	0.91
66	1.78	0.91	1.55	0.92	1.26	0.92	1.35	0.92	1.15	0.91
67	1.85	0.92	1.61	0.93	1.31	0.92	1.40	0.92	1.20	0.92
68	1.91	0.92	1.67	0.95	1.36	0.94	1.45	0.93	1.24	0.92
69	1.97	0.93	1.73	0.95	1.40	0.94	1.50	0.96	1.29	0.94
70	2.04	0.95	1.78	0.96	1.45	0.96	1.55	0.96	1.34	0.95
71	2.10	0.95	1.84	0.97	1.50	0.96	1.60	0.96	1.39	0.95
72	2.17	0.97	1.90	0.97	1.55	0.96	1.65	0.96	1.43	0.96
73	2.23	0.97	1.96	0.98	1.60	0.97	1.70	0.97	1.48	0.96
74	2.30	0.97	2.01	0.98	1.64	0.97	1.75	0.97	1.53	0.96
75	2.36	0.98	2.07	0.98	1.69	0.98	1.80	0.98	1.58	0.96

Table A–7. Personality Inventory for DSM-5—Self-Report Form (100 item) normative tables: domain scales *(continued)*

T	Negative affect		Detachment		Antagonism		Disinhibition		Psychoticism	
	Raw	Percentile	Raw	Percentile	Raw	Percentile	Raw	Percentile	Raw	Percentile
76	2.42	0.98	2.13	0.98	1.74	0.98	1.85	0.98	1.62	0.97
77	2.49	0.98	2.19	0.98	1.79	0.98	1.90	0.98	1.67	0.98
78	2.55	0.99	2.24	0.98	1.83	0.98	1.95	0.98	1.72	0.98
79	2.62	1.00	2.30	0.99	1.88	0.98	2.00	0.98	1.77	0.98
80	2.68	1.00	2.36	0.99	1.93	0.98	2.05	0.99	1.82	0.98
81	2.75	1.00	2.42	0.99	1.98	0.98	2.10	0.99	1.86	0.99
82	2.81	1.00	2.47	0.99	2.03	0.99	2.15	0.99	1.91	0.99
83	2.87	1.00	2.53	1.00	2.07	0.99	2.20	0.99	1.96	0.99
84	2.94	1.00	2.59	1.00	2.12	0.99	2.25	0.99	2.01	0.99
85	3.00	1.00	2.65	1.00	2.17	1.00	2.29	1.00	2.05	0.99
86	3.07	1.00	2.70	1.00	2.22	1.00	2.34	1.00	2.10	0.99
87	3.13	1.00	2.76	1.00	2.26	1.00	2.39	1.00	2.15	0.99
88	3.20	1.00	2.82	1.00	2.31	1.00	2.44	1.00	2.20	0.99
89	3.26	1.00	2.88	1.00	2.36	1.00	2.49	1.00	2.25	0.99
90	3.32	1.00	2.93	1.00	2.41	1.00	2.54	1.00	2.29	1.00

Table A–8. Personality Inventory for DSM-5—Self-Report Form (100 item) normative tables: trait scales

T	Anhedonia		Anxiousness		Attention seeking		Callousness		Deceitfulness	
	Raw	Percentile	Raw	Percentile	Raw	Percentile	Raw	Percentile	Raw	Percentile
30	0.00	0.00	0.00	0.00	0.00	0.00	0.00	0.00	0.00	0.00
31	0.00	0.00	0.00	0.00	0.00	0.00	0.00	0.00	0.00	0.00
32	0.00	0.00	0.00	0.00	0.00	0.00	0.00	0.00	0.00	0.00
33	0.00	0.00	0.00	0.00	0.00	0.00	0.00	0.00	0.00	0.00
34	0.00	0.00	0.00	0.00	0.00	0.00	0.00	0.00	0.00	0.00
35	0.00	0.00	0.00	0.00	0.00	0.00	0.00	0.00	0.00	0.00
36	0.00	0.00	0.00	0.00	0.00	0.00	0.00	0.00	0.00	0.00
37	0.00	0.00	0.00	0.00	0.00	0.00	0.00	0.00	0.00	0.00
38	0.00	0.00	0.00	0.00	0.00	0.00	0.00	0.00	0.00	0.00
39	0.00	0.00	0.00	0.00	0.00	0.00	0.00	0.00	0.00	0.00
40	0.00	0.00	0.07	0.25	0.02	0.27	0.00	0.00	0.00	0.00
41	0.00	0.00	0.15	0.25	0.09	0.27	0.00	0.00	0.00	0.00
42	0.03	0.39	0.23	0.25	0.17	0.27	0.00	0.00	0.00	0.00
43	0.10	0.39	0.31	0.37	0.24	0.27	0.00	0.00	0.00	0.00
44	0.16	0.39	0.39	0.37	0.31	0.40	0.01	0.58	0.03	0.57
45	0.23	0.39	0.48	0.37	0.38	0.40	0.06	0.58	0.08	0.57

Table A–8. Personality Inventory for DSM-5—Self-Report Form (100 item) normative tables: trait scales (continued)

T	Anhedonia		Anxiousness		Attention seeking		Callousness		Deceitfulness	
	Raw	Percentile	Raw	Percentile	Raw	Percentile	Raw	Percentile	Raw	Percentile
46	0.30	0.54	0.56	0.50	0.45	0.40	0.11	0.58	0.13	0.57
47	0.37	0.55	0.64	0.50	0.52	0.52	0.16	0.58	0.19	0.57
48	0.44	0.55	0.72	0.51	0.60	0.52	0.21	0.58	0.24	0.57
49	0.50	0.65	0.80	0.59	0.67	0.52	0.26	0.76	0.29	0.72
50	0.57	0.65	0.88	0.59	0.74	0.52	0.31	0.76	0.34	0.72
51	0.64	0.65	0.96	0.59	0.81	0.62	0.36	0.77	0.39	0.72
52	0.71	0.66	1.04	0.69	0.88	0.62	0.42	0.77	0.44	0.72
53	0.77	0.74	1.13	0.69	0.95	0.62	0.47	0.77	0.49	0.72
54	0.84	0.74	1.21	0.69	1.02	0.73	0.52	0.85	0.54	0.83
55	0.91	0.74	1.29	0.77	1.10	0.73	0.57	0.85	0.59	0.83
56	0.98	0.74	1.37	0.77	1.17	0.73	0.62	0.85	0.64	0.83
57	1.04	0.82	1.45	0.77	1.24	0.73	0.67	0.85	0.69	0.83
58	1.11	0.82	1.53	0.83	1.31	0.79	0.72	0.85	0.74	0.83
59	1.18	0.82	1.61	0.83	1.38	0.80	0.77	0.90	0.80	0.90
60	1.25	0.82	1.70	0.84	1.45	0.80	0.82	0.90	0.85	0.90
61	1.32	0.88	1.78	0.89	1.52	0.86	0.87	0.90	0.90	0.90

Table A–8. Personality Inventory for DSM-5—Self-Report Form (100 item) normative tables: trait scales (*continued*)

T	Anhedonia Raw	Anhedonia Percentile	Anxiousness Raw	Anxiousness Percentile	Attention seeking Raw	Attention seeking Percentile	Callousness Raw	Callousness Percentile	Deceitfulness Raw	Deceitfulness Percentile
62	1.38	0.88	1.86	0.89	1.60	0.86	0.92	0.90	0.95	0.90
63	1.45	0.88	1.94	0.89	1.67	0.86	0.98	0.90	1.00	0.90
64	1.52	0.92	2.02	0.93	1.74	0.86	1.03	0.94	1.05	0.94
65	1.59	0.92	2.10	0.93	1.81	0.91	1.08	0.94	1.10	0.94
66	1.65	0.92	2.18	0.93	1.88	0.91	1.13	0.94	1.15	0.94
67	1.72	0.92	2.26	0.95	1.95	0.91	1.18	0.94	1.20	0.94
68	1.79	0.94	2.35	0.95	2.03	0.97	1.23	0.94	1.25	0.96
69	1.86	0.94	2.43	0.95	2.10	0.97	1.28	0.96	1.30	0.96
70	1.92	0.94	2.51	0.97	2.17	0.97	1.33	0.96	1.35	0.97
71	1.99	0.94	2.59	0.97	2.24	0.97	1.38	0.96	1.40	0.97
72	2.06	0.97	2.67	0.98	2.31	0.98	1.43	0.96	1.46	0.97
73	2.13	0.97	2.75	0.99	2.38	0.98	1.48	0.96	1.51	0.98
74	2.19	0.97	2.83	0.99	2.45	0.98	1.54	0.97	1.56	0.98
75	2.26	0.98	2.92	0.99	2.53	0.99	1.59	0.97	1.61	0.98
76	2.33	0.98	3.00	0.99	2.60	0.99	1.64	0.97	1.66	0.98
77	2.40	0.98	3.08	1.00	2.67	0.99	1.69	0.97	1.71	0.98

Table A–8. Personality Inventory for DSM-5—Self-Report Form (100 item) normative tables: trait scales (continued)

T	Anhedonia		Anxiousness		Attention seeking		Callousness		Deceitfulness	
	Raw	Percentile	Raw	Percentile	Raw	Percentile	Raw	Percentile	Raw	Percentile
78	2.47	0.98	3.16	1.00	2.74	0.99	1.74	0.97	1.76	0.99
79	2.53	0.99	3.24	1.00	2.81	1.00	1.79	0.98	1.81	0.99
80	2.60	0.99	3.32	1.00	2.88	1.00	1.84	0.98	1.86	0.99
81	2.67	0.99	3.40	1.00	2.95	1.00	1.89	0.98	1.91	0.99
82	2.74	0.99	3.48	1.00	3.03	1.00	1.94	0.98	1.96	0.99
83	2.80	1.00	3.57	1.00	3.10	1.00	1.99	0.98	2.01	0.99
84	2.87	1.00	3.65	1.00	3.17	1.00	2.04	0.99	2.07	0.99
85	2.94	1.00	3.73	1.00	3.24	1.00	2.10	0.99	2.12	0.99
86	3.01	1.00	3.81	1.00	3.31	1.00	2.15	0.99	2.17	0.99
87	3.07	1.00	3.89	1.00	3.38	1.00	2.20	0.99	2.22	0.99
88	3.14	1.00	3.97	1.00	3.45	1.00	2.25	0.99	2.27	0.99
89	3.21	1.00	4.00	1.00	3.53	1.00	2.30	1.00	2.32	0.99
90	3.28	1.00	4.00	1.00	3.60	1.00	2.35	1.00	2.37	0.99
91	3.35	1.00	4.00	1.00	3.67	1.00	2.40	1.00	2.42	0.99
92	3.41	1.00	4.00	1.00	3.74	1.00	2.45	1.00	2.47	0.99
93	3.48	1.00	4.00	1.00	3.81	1.00	2.50	1.00	2.52	1.00

Table A–8. Personality Inventory for DSM-5—Self-Report Form (100 item) normative tables: trait scales *(continued)*

T	Anhedonia Raw	Anhedonia Percentile	Anxiousness Raw	Anxiousness Percentile	Attention seeking Raw	Attention seeking Percentile	Callousness Raw	Callousness Percentile	Deceitfulness Raw	Deceitfulness Percentile
94	3.55	1.00	4.00	1.00	3.88	1.00	2.55	1.00	2.57	1.00
95	3.62	1.00	4.00	1.00	3.96	1.00	2.60	1.00	2.62	1.00
96	3.68	1.00	4.00	1.00	4.00	1.00	2.66	1.00	2.67	1.00
97	3.75	1.00	4.00	1.00	4.00	1.00	2.71	1.00	2.73	1.00
98	3.82	1.00	4.00	1.00	4.00	1.00	2.76	1.00	2.78	1.00
99	3.89	1.00	4.00	1.00	4.00	1.00	2.81	1.00	2.83	1.00
100	3.95	1.00	4.00	1.00	4.00	1.00	2.86	1.00	2.88	1.00

T	Depressivity Raw	Depressivity Percentile	Distractibility Raw	Distractibility Percentile	Eccentricity Raw	Eccentricity Percentile	Emotional lability Raw	Emotional lability Percentile	Grandiosity Raw	Grandiosity Percentile
30	0.00	0.00	0.00	0.00	0.00	0.00	0.00	0.00	0.00	0.00
31	0.00	0.00	0.00	0.00	0.00	0.00	0.00	0.00	0.00	0.00
32	0.00	0.00	0.00	0.00	0.00	0.00	0.00	0.00	0.00	0.00
33	0.00	0.00	0.00	0.00	0.00	0.00	0.00	0.00	0.00	0.00
34	0.00	0.00	0.00	0.00	0.00	0.00	0.00	0.00	0.00	0.00
35	0.00	0.00	0.00	0.00	0.00	0.00	0.00	0.00	0.00	0.00

Table A–8. Personality Inventory for DSM-5—Self-Report Form (100 item) normative tables: trait scales (*continued*)

T	Depressivity		Distractibility		Eccentricity		Emotional lability		Grandiosity	
	Raw	Percentile	Raw	Percentile	Raw	Percentile	Raw	Percentile	Raw	Percentile
36	0.00	0.00	0.00	0.00	0.00	0.00	0.00	0.00	0.00	0.00
37	0.00	0.00	0.00	0.00	0.00	0.00	0.00	0.00	0.00	0.00
38	0.00	0.00	0.00	0.00	0.00	0.00	0.00	0.00	0.00	0.00
39	0.00	0.00	0.00	0.00	0.00	0.00	0.00	0.00	0.00	0.00
40	0.00	0.00	0.00	0.00	0.00	0.00	0.00	0.00	0.00	0.00
41	0.00	0.00	0.06	0.30	0.00	0.00	0.00	0.00	0.00	0.38
42	0.00	0.00	0.14	0.30	0.00	0.00	0.04	0.38	0.06	0.38
43	0.00	0.00	0.21	0.30	0.07	0.43	0.12	0.38	0.12	0.38
44	0.00	0.00	0.29	0.43	0.15	0.43	0.19	0.38	0.18	0.38
45	0.00	0.68	0.37	0.44	0.23	0.43	0.26	0.51	0.24	0.38
46	0.06	0.68	0.44	0.44	0.31	0.57	0.33	0.51	0.29	0.55
47	0.12	0.68	0.52	0.55	0.39	0.57	0.41	0.51	0.35	0.55
48	0.18	0.68	0.59	0.55	0.47	0.57	0.48	0.51	0.41	0.55
49	0.23	0.68	0.67	0.56	0.54	0.66	0.55	0.63	0.47	0.55
50	0.29	0.78	0.74	0.56	0.62	0.66	0.63	0.63	0.53	0.70
51	0.35	0.78	0.82	0.64	0.70	0.66	0.70	0.63	0.59	0.70

Table A–8. Personality Inventory for DSM-5—Self-Report Form (100 item) normative tables: trait scales *(continued)*

T	Depressivity		Distractibility		Eccentricity		Emotional lability		Grandiosity	
	Raw	Percentile	Raw	Percentile	Raw	Percentile	Raw	Percentile	Raw	Percentile
52	0.41	0.78	0.89	0.64	0.78	0.73	0.77	0.72	0.64	0.70
53	0.46	0.78	0.97	0.64	0.86	0.73	0.84	0.72	0.70	0.70
54	0.52	0.83	1.04	0.75	0.94	0.73	0.92	0.72	0.76	0.80
55	0.58	0.83	1.12	0.75	1.02	0.79	0.99	0.72	0.82	0.80
56	0.64	0.83	1.20	0.75	1.10	0.79	1.06	0.80	0.88	0.80
57	0.69	0.83	1.27	0.83	1.17	0.79	1.14	0.80	0.93	0.80
58	0.75	0.87	1.35	0.83	1.25	0.85	1.21	0.80	0.99	0.80
59	0.81	0.87	1.42	0.83	1.33	0.85	1.28	0.87	1.05	0.87
60	0.87	0.87	1.50	0.83	1.41	0.85	1.35	0.87	1.11	0.87
61	0.92	0.87	1.57	0.88	1.49	0.85	1.43	0.87	1.17	0.87
62	0.98	0.87	1.65	0.88	1.57	0.89	1.50	0.91	1.23	0.87
63	1.04	0.92	1.72	0.88	1.65	0.89	1.57	0.91	1.28	0.92
64	1.10	0.92	1.80	0.92	1.73	0.90	1.65	0.91	1.34	0.92
65	1.15	0.92	1.88	0.92	1.80	0.93	1.72	0.91	1.40	0.92
66	1.21	0.92	1.95	0.92	1.88	0.93	1.79	0.93	1.46	0.92
67	1.27	0.94	2.03	0.96	1.96	0.93	1.86	0.93	1.52	0.95

Table A–8. Personality Inventory for DSM-5—Self-Report Form (100 item) normative tables: trait scales (continued)

T	Depressivity		Distractibility		Eccentricity		Emotional lability		Grandiosity	
	Raw	Percentile	Raw	Percentile	Raw	Percentile	Raw	Percentile	Raw	Percentile
68	1.33	0.94	2.10	0.96	2.04	0.96	1.94	0.93	1.57	0.95
69	1.38	0.94	2.18	0.96	2.12	0.96	2.01	0.96	1.63	0.95
70	1.44	0.94	2.25	0.97	2.20	0.96	2.08	0.96	1.69	0.95
71	1.50	0.94	2.33	0.97	2.28	0.98	2.16	0.96	1.75	0.95
72	1.56	0.96	2.40	0.98	2.36	0.98	2.23	0.96	1.81	0.97
73	1.61	0.96	2.48	0.98	2.43	0.98	2.30	0.97	1.87	0.97
74	1.67	0.96	2.55	0.99	2.51	0.98	2.37	0.97	1.92	0.97
75	1.73	0.96	2.63	0.99	2.59	0.98	2.45	0.97	1.98	0.97
76	1.79	0.97	2.71	0.99	2.67	0.98	2.52	0.98	2.04	0.99
77	1.84	0.97	2.78	0.99	2.75	0.98	2.59	0.98	2.10	0.99
78	1.90	0.97	2.86	0.99	2.83	0.99	2.67	0.98	2.16	0.99
79	1.96	0.97	2.93	0.99	2.91	0.99	2.74	0.98	2.22	0.99
80	2.02	0.98	3.01	1.00	2.99	0.99	2.81	0.99	2.27	1.00
81	2.07	0.98	3.08	1.00	3.06	1.00	2.88	0.99	2.33	1.00
82	2.13	0.98	3.16	1.00	3.14	1.00	2.96	0.99	2.39	1.00
83	2.19	0.98	3.23	1.00	3.22	1.00	3.03	1.00	2.45	1.00

Table A–8. Personality Inventory for DSM-5—Self-Report Form (100 item) normative tables: trait scales *(continued)*

T	Depressivity		Distractibility		Eccentricity		Emotional lability		Grandiosity	
	Raw	Percentile	Raw	Percentile	Raw	Percentile	Raw	Percentile	Raw	Percentile
84	2.25	0.98	3.31	1.00	3.30	1.00	3.10	1.00	2.51	1.00
85	2.30	0.99	3.39	1.00	3.38	1.00	3.18	1.00	2.56	1.00
86	2.36	0.99	3.46	1.00	3.46	1.00	3.25	1.00	2.62	1.00
87	2.42	0.99	3.54	1.00	3.54	1.00	3.32	1.00	2.68	1.00
88	2.48	0.99	3.61	1.00	3.62	1.00	3.39	1.00	2.74	1.00
89	2.53	1.00	3.69	1.00	3.70	1.00	3.47	1.00	2.80	1.00
90	2.59	1.00	3.76	1.00	3.77	1.00	3.54	1.00	2.86	1.00
91	2.65	1.00	3.84	1.00	3.85	1.00	3.61	1.00	2.91	1.00
92	2.71	1.00	3.91	1.00	3.93	1.00	3.69	1.00	2.97	1.00
93	2.76	1.00	3.99	1.00	4.00	1.00	3.76	1.00	3.03	1.00
94	2.82	1.00	4.00	1.00	4.00	1.00	3.83	1.00	3.09	1.00
95	2.88	1.00	4.00	1.00	4.00	1.00	3.90	1.00	3.15	1.00
96	2.94	1.00	4.00	1.00	4.00	1.00	3.98	1.00	3.20	1.00
97	2.99	1.00	4.00	1.00	4.00	1.00	4.00	1.00	3.26	1.00
98	3.05	1.00	4.00	1.00	4.00	1.00	4.00	1.00	3.32	1.00
99	3.11	1.00	4.00	1.00	4.00	1.00	4.00	1.00	3.38	1.00
100	3.17	1.00	4.00	1.00	4.00	1.00	4.00	1.00	3.44	1.00

Table A–8. Personality Inventory for DSM-5—Self-Report Form (100 item) normative tables: trait scales *(continued)*

T	Hostility		Impulsivity		Intimacy avoidance		Irresponsibility		Manipulativeness	
	Raw	Percentile	Raw	Percentile	Raw	Percentile	Raw	Percentile	Raw	Percentile
30	0.00	0.00	0.00	0.00	0.00	0.00	0.00	0.00	0.00	0.00
31	0.00	0.00	0.00	0.00	0.00	0.00	0.00	0.00	0.00	0.00
32	0.00	0.00	0.00	0.00	0.00	0.00	0.00	0.00	0.00	0.00
33	0.00	0.00	0.00	0.00	0.00	0.00	0.00	0.00	0.00	0.00
34	0.00	0.00	0.00	0.00	0.00	0.00	0.00	0.00	0.00	0.00
35	0.00	0.00	0.00	0.00	0.00	0.00	0.00	0.00	0.00	0.00
36	0.00	0.00	0.00	0.00	0.00	0.00	0.00	0.00	0.00	0.00
37	0.00	0.00	0.00	0.00	0.00	0.00	0.00	0.00	0.00	0.00
38	0.00	0.00	0.00	0.00	0.00	0.00	0.00	0.00	0.00	0.00
39	0.00	0.00	0.00	0.00	0.00	0.00	0.00	0.00	0.00	0.00
40	0.00	0.00	0.01	0.28	0.00	0.00	0.00	0.00	0.02	0.26
41	0.05	0.29	0.07	0.28	0.00	0.00	0.00	0.00	0.08	0.26
42	0.12	0.29	0.14	0.28	0.00	0.00	0.00	0.00	0.14	0.26
43	0.19	0.29	0.21	0.28	0.05	0.44	0.00	0.00	0.20	0.26
44	0.26	0.42	0.27	0.44	0.12	0.44	0.02	0.58	0.26	0.43
45	0.33	0.42	0.34	0.44	0.19	0.44	0.06	0.58	0.32	0.43
46	0.40	0.43	0.40	0.44	0.26	0.56	0.10	0.58	0.38	0.43

Table A–8. Personality Inventory for DSM-5—Self-Report Form (100 item) normative tables: trait scales *(continued)*

T	Hostility		Impulsivity		Intimacy avoidance		Irresponsibility		Manipulativeness	
	Raw	Percentile	Raw	Percentile	Raw	Percentile	Raw	Percentile	Raw	Percentile
47	0.47	0.43	0.47	0.44	0.34	0.57	0.15	0.58	0.44	0.43
48	0.54	0.56	0.53	0.58	0.41	0.57	0.19	0.58	0.50	0.61
49	0.61	0.56	0.60	0.58	0.48	0.57	0.23	0.58	0.56	0.61
50	0.68	0.56	0.66	0.58	0.55	0.69	0.27	0.75	0.62	0.61
51	0.75	0.56	0.73	0.59	0.63	0.69	0.31	0.75	0.68	0.61
52	0.82	0.69	0.79	0.69	0.70	0.69	0.36	0.75	0.74	0.61
53	0.89	0.69	0.86	0.69	0.77	0.77	0.40	0.75	0.81	0.73
54	0.96	0.69	0.92	0.69	0.84	0.77	0.44	0.75	0.87	0.73
55	1.03	0.77	0.99	0.69	0.91	0.77	0.48	0.75	0.93	0.73
56	1.10	0.77	1.05	0.81	0.99	0.77	0.53	0.87	0.99	0.73
57	1.17	0.77	1.12	0.81	1.06	0.82	0.57	0.87	1.05	0.84
58	1.24	0.77	1.18	0.81	1.13	0.82	0.61	0.87	1.11	0.84
59	1.31	0.86	1.25	0.81	1.20	0.82	0.65	0.87	1.17	0.84
60	1.38	0.86	1.31	0.86	1.28	0.88	0.70	0.87	1.23	0.84
61	1.45	0.86	1.38	0.86	1.35	0.88	0.74	0.87	1.29	0.90
62	1.52	0.91	1.44	0.86	1.42	0.88	0.78	0.93	1.35	0.90

Table A–8. Personality Inventory for DSM-5—Self-Report Form (100 item) normative tables: trait scales (continued)

T	Hostility		Impulsivity		Intimacy avoidance		Irresponsibility		Manipulativeness	
	Raw	Percentile	Raw	Percentile	Raw	Percentile	Raw	Percentile	Raw	Percentile
63	1.59	0.91	1.51	0.91	1.49	0.88	0.82	0.93	1.41	0.90
64	1.66	0.91	1.57	0.91	1.56	0.91	0.87	0.93	1.47	0.90
65	1.73	0.91	1.64	0.91	1.64	0.91	0.91	0.93	1.53	0.94
66	1.80	0.94	1.70	0.91	1.71	0.91	0.95	0.93	1.59	0.94
67	1.87	0.94	1.77	0.94	1.78	0.93	0.99	0.93	1.65	0.94
68	1.94	0.94	1.84	0.94	1.85	0.93	1.03	0.96	1.71	0.94
69	2.01	0.96	1.90	0.94	1.93	0.93	1.08	0.96	1.78	0.97
70	2.08	0.96	1.97	0.94	2.00	0.93	1.12	0.96	1.84	0.97
71	2.15	0.96	2.03	0.98	2.07	0.96	1.16	0.96	1.90	0.97
72	2.22	0.96	2.10	0.98	2.14	0.96	1.20	0.96	1.96	0.97
73	2.29	0.98	2.16	0.98	2.22	0.96	1.25	0.96	2.02	0.98
74	2.36	0.98	2.23	0.98	2.29	0.97	1.29	0.97	2.08	0.98
75	2.43	0.98	2.29	0.99	2.36	0.97	1.33	0.97	2.14	0.98
76	2.50	0.98	2.36	0.99	2.43	0.97	1.37	0.97	2.20	0.98
77	2.57	0.99	2.42	0.99	2.50	0.98	1.42	0.97	2.26	0.99
78	2.64	0.99	2.49	0.99	2.58	0.98	1.46	0.97	2.32	0.99

Table A–8. Personality Inventory for DSM-5—Self-Report Form (100 item) normative tables: trait scales *(continued)*

T	Hostility		Impulsivity		Intimacy avoidance		Irresponsibility		Manipulativeness	
	Raw	Percentile	Raw	Percentile	Raw	Percentile	Raw	Percentile	Raw	Percentile
79	2.71	0.99	2.55	0.99	2.65	0.98	1.50	0.99	2.38	0.99
80	2.78	1.00	2.62	0.99	2.72	0.98	1.54	0.99	2.44	0.99
81	2.85	1.00	2.68	0.99	2.79	0.99	1.59	0.99	2.50	0.99
82	2.92	1.00	2.75	0.99	2.87	0.99	1.63	0.99	2.56	0.99
83	2.99	1.00	2.81	1.00	2.94	0.99	1.67	0.99	2.62	0.99
84	3.06	1.00	2.88	1.00	3.01	1.00	1.71	0.99	2.68	0.99
85	3.13	1.00	2.94	1.00	3.08	1.00	1.76	0.99	2.74	0.99
86	3.20	1.00	3.01	1.00	3.15	1.00	1.80	0.99	2.81	0.99
87	3.27	1.00	3.07	1.00	3.23	1.00	1.84	0.99	2.87	0.99
88	3.34	1.00	3.14	1.00	3.30	1.00	1.88	0.99	2.93	0.99
89	3.41	1.00	3.20	1.00	3.37	1.00	1.92	0.99	2.99	0.99
90	3.48	1.00	3.27	1.00	3.44	1.00	1.97	0.99	3.05	1.00
91	3.55	1.00	3.34	1.00	3.52	1.00	2.01	1.00	3.11	1.00
92	3.62	1.00	3.40	1.00	3.59	1.00	2.05	1.00	3.17	1.00
93	3.69	1.00	3.47	1.00	3.66	1.00	2.09	1.00	3.23	1.00
94	3.76	1.00	3.53	1.00	3.73	1.00	2.14	1.00	3.29	1.00

Table A–8. Personality Inventory for DSM-5—Self-Report Form (100 item) normative tables: trait scales (continued)

T	Hostility		Impulsivity		Intimacy avoidance		Irresponsibility		Manipulativeness	
	Raw	Percentile	Raw	Percentile	Raw	Percentile	Raw	Percentile	Raw	Percentile
95	3.83	1.00	3.60	1.00	3.80	1.00	2.18	1.00	3.35	1.00
96	3.90	1.00	3.66	1.00	3.88	1.00	2.22	1.00	3.41	1.00
97	3.97	1.00	3.73	1.00	3.95	1.00	2.26	1.00	3.47	1.00
98	4.00	1.00	3.79	1.00	4.00	1.00	2.31	1.00	3.53	1.00
99	4.00	1.00	3.86	1.00	4.00	1.00	2.35	1.00	3.59	1.00
100	4.00	1.00	3.92	1.00	4.00	1.00	2.39	1.00	3.65	1.00

T	Perceptual dysregulation		Perseveration		Restricted affectivity		Rigid perfectionism		Risk taking	
	Raw	Percentile	Raw	Percentile	Raw	Percentile	Raw	Percentile	Raw	Percentile
30	0.00	0.00	0.00	0.00	0.00	0.00	0.00	0.00	0.00	0.00
31	0.00	0.00	0.00	0.00	0.00	0.00	0.00	0.00	0.00	0.00
32	0.00	0.00	0.00	0.00	0.00	0.00	0.00	0.00	0.00	0.00
33	0.00	0.00	0.00	0.00	0.00	0.00	0.00	0.00	0.00	0.00
34	0.00	0.00	0.00	0.00	0.00	0.00	0.00	0.00	0.00	0.00
35	0.00	0.00	0.00	0.00	0.00	0.00	0.00	0.00	0.00	0.00

Table A–8. Personality Inventory for DSM-5—Self-Report Form (100 item) normative tables: trait scales *(continued)*

T	Perceptual dysregulation		Perseveration		Restricted affectivity		Rigid perfectionism		Risk taking	
	Raw	Percentile	Raw	Percentile	Raw	Percentile	Raw	Percentile	Raw	Percentile
36	0.00	0.00	0.00	0.00	0.05	0.10	0.00	0.00	0.00	0.00
37	0.00	0.00	0.00	0.00	0.11	0.10	0.00	0.00	0.00	0.00
38	0.00	0.00	0.00	0.00	0.18	0.10	0.00	0.00	0.00	0.00
39	0.00	0.00	0.00	0.00	0.24	0.10	0.00	0.00	0.00	0.00
40	0.00	0.00	0.02	0.27	0.31	0.19	0.05	0.27	0.00	0.00
41	0.00	0.00	0.08	0.27	0.37	0.19	0.13	0.27	0.00	0.00
42	0.00	0.00	0.15	0.27	0.44	0.19	0.20	0.27	0.00	0.41
43	0.00	0.00	0.21	0.41	0.50	0.31	0.28	0.38	0.06	0.41
44	0.00	0.00	0.28	0.42	0.57	0.31	0.35	0.39	0.12	0.41
45	0.00	0.00	0.35	0.42	0.63	0.31	0.42	0.39	0.18	0.41
46	0.02	0.77	0.41	0.42	0.70	0.31	0.50	0.39	0.23	0.41
47	0.06	0.77	0.48	0.42	0.76	0.48	0.57	0.50	0.29	0.58
48	0.09	0.77	0.55	0.56	0.83	0.48	0.65	0.50	0.35	0.58
49	0.12	0.77	0.61	0.56	0.89	0.48	0.72	0.50	0.40	0.58
50	0.16	0.77	0.68	0.56	0.95	0.48	0.80	0.62	0.46	0.58

Table A–8. Personality Inventory for DSM-5—Self-Report Form (100 item) normative tables: trait scales (continued)

T	Perceptual dysregulation		Perseveration		Restricted affectivity		Rigid perfectionism		Risk taking	
	Raw	Percentile	Raw	Percentile	Raw	Percentile	Raw	Percentile	Raw	Percentile
51	0.19	0.77	0.74	0.56	1.02	0.64	0.87	0.62	0.52	0.72
52	0.23	0.77	0.81	0.69	1.08	0.64	0.94	0.62	0.58	0.72
53	0.26	0.86	0.88	0.69	1.15	0.64	1.02	0.73	0.63	0.72
54	0.29	0.86	0.94	0.69	1.21	0.64	1.09	0.73	0.69	0.72
55	0.33	0.86	1.01	0.81	1.28	0.76	1.17	0.73	0.75	0.72
56	0.36	0.87	1.07	0.81	1.34	0.76	1.24	0.73	0.81	0.82
57	0.40	0.87	1.14	0.81	1.41	0.76	1.32	0.80	0.86	0.82
58	0.43	0.87	1.21	0.81	1.47	0.76	1.39	0.80	0.92	0.82
59	0.46	0.87	1.27	0.87	1.54	0.84	1.46	0.80	0.98	0.82
60	0.50	0.87	1.34	0.87	1.60	0.84	1.54	0.85	1.04	0.87
61	0.53	0.91	1.41	0.87	1.67	0.84	1.61	0.85	1.09	0.87
62	0.57	0.91	1.47	0.87	1.73	0.84	1.69	0.85	1.15	0.87
63	0.60	0.91	1.54	0.92	1.80	0.90	1.76	0.92	1.21	0.87
64	0.63	0.91	1.60	0.92	1.86	0.90	1.84	0.92	1.26	0.93
65	0.67	0.92	1.67	0.92	1.92	0.90	1.91	0.92	1.32	0.93

Table A–8. Personality Inventory for DSM-5—Self-Report Form (100 item) normative tables: trait scales *(continued)*

T	Perceptual dysregulation		Perseveration		Restricted affectivity		Rigid perfectionism		Risk taking	
	Raw	Percentile	Raw	Percentile	Raw	Percentile	Raw	Percentile	Raw	Percentile
66	0.70	0.92	1.74	0.92	1.99	0.90	1.98	0.92	1.38	0.93
67	0.74	0.92	1.80	0.95	2.05	0.96	2.06	0.95	1.44	0.93
68	0.77	0.93	1.87	0.95	2.12	0.96	2.13	0.95	1.49	0.93
69	0.81	0.93	1.93	0.95	2.18	0.96	2.21	0.95	1.55	0.96
70	0.84	0.93	2.00	0.98	2.25	0.96	2.28	0.98	1.61	0.96
71	0.87	0.93	2.07	0.98	2.31	0.98	2.35	0.98	1.67	0.96
72	0.91	0.93	2.13	0.98	2.38	0.98	2.43	0.98	1.72	0.96
73	0.94	0.93	2.20	0.98	2.44	0.98	2.50	0.98	1.78	0.97
74	0.98	0.93	2.27	0.99	2.51	0.99	2.58	0.98	1.84	0.97
75	1.01	0.97	2.33	0.99	2.57	0.99	2.65	0.98	1.89	0.97
76	1.04	0.97	2.40	0.99	2.64	0.99	2.73	0.98	1.95	0.97
77	1.08	0.97	2.46	0.99	2.70	0.99	2.80	0.99	2.01	0.98
78	1.11	0.97	2.53	0.99	2.77	1.00	2.87	0.99	2.07	0.98
79	1.15	0.97	2.60	0.99	2.83	1.00	2.95	0.99	2.12	0.98
80	1.18	0.97	2.66	0.99	2.89	1.00	3.02	1.00	2.18	0.98

Table A–8. Personality Inventory for DSM-5—Self-Report Form (100 item) normative tables: trait scales (continued)

T	Perceptual dysregulation		Perseveration		Restricted affectivity		Rigid perfectionism		Risk taking	
	Raw	Percentile	Raw	Percentile	Raw	Percentile	Raw	Percentile	Raw	Percentile
81	1.21	0.97	2.73	0.99	2.96	1.00	3.10	1.00	2.24	0.98
82	1.25	0.97	2.79	1.00	3.02	1.00	3.17	1.00	2.30	0.99
83	1.28	0.98	2.86	1.00	3.09	1.00	3.25	1.00	2.35	0.99
84	1.32	0.98	2.93	1.00	3.15	1.00	3.32	1.00	2.41	0.99
85	1.35	0.98	2.99	1.00	3.22	1.00	3.39	1.00	2.47	0.99
86	1.38	0.98	3.06	1.00	3.28	1.00	3.47	1.00	2.52	0.99
87	1.42	0.98	3.13	1.00	3.35	1.00	3.54	1.00	2.58	0.99
88	1.45	0.98	3.19	1.00	3.41	1.00	3.62	1.00	2.64	0.99
89	1.49	0.98	3.26	1.00	3.48	1.00	3.69	1.00	2.70	0.99
90	1.52	1.00	3.32	1.00	3.54	1.00	3.76	1.00	2.75	1.00
91	1.55	1.00	3.39	1.00	3.61	1.00	3.84	1.00	2.81	1.00
92	1.59	1.00	3.46	1.00	3.67	1.00	3.91	1.00	2.87	1.00
93	1.62	1.00	3.52	1.00	3.74	1.00	3.99	1.00	2.93	1.00
94	1.66	1.00	3.59	1.00	3.80	1.00	4.00	1.00	2.98	1.00
95	1.69	1.00	3.66	1.00	3.86	1.00	4.00	1.00	3.04	1.00

Table A–8. Personality Inventory for DSM-5—Self-Report Form (100 item) normative tables: trait scales *(continued)*

T	Perceptual dysregulation		Perseveration		Restricted affectivity		Rigid perfectionism		Risk taking	
	Raw	Percentile	Raw	Percentile	Raw	Percentile	Raw	Percentile	Raw	Percentile
96	1.73	1.00	3.72	1.00	3.93	1.00	4.00	1.00	3.10	1.00
97	1.76	1.00	3.79	1.00	3.99	1.00	4.00	1.00	3.15	1.00
98	1.79	1.00	3.85	1.00	4.00	1.00	4.00	1.00	3.21	1.00
99	1.83	1.00	3.92	1.00	4.00	1.00	4.00	1.00	3.27	1.00
100	1.86	1.00	3.99	1.00	4.00	1.00	4.00	1.00	3.33	1.00

T	Separation insecurity		Submissiveness		Suspiciousness		Unusual beliefs and experiences		Withdrawal	
	Raw	Percentile	Raw	Percentile	Raw	Percentile	Raw	Percentile	Raw	Percentile
30	0.00	0.00	0.00	0.00	0.00	0.00	0.00	0.00	0.00	0.00
31	0.00	0.00	0.00	0.00	0.00	0.00	0.00	0.00	0.00	0.00
32	0.00	0.00	0.00	0.00	0.00	0.00	0.00	0.00	0.00	0.00
33	0.00	0.00	0.00	0.00	0.00	0.00	0.00	0.00	0.00	0.00
34	0.00	0.00	0.01	0.07	0.00	0.00	0.00	0.00	0.00	0.00
35	0.00	0.00	0.08	0.07	0.00	0.00	0.00	0.00	0.00	0.00
36	0.00	0.00	0.15	0.07	0.00	0.00	0.00	0.00	0.00	0.00

Table A–8. Personality Inventory for DSM-5—Self-Report Form (100 item) normative tables: trait scales (continued)

T	Separation insecurity		Submissiveness		Suspiciousness		Unusual beliefs and experiences		Withdrawal	
	Raw	Percentile	Raw	Percentile	Raw	Percentile	Raw	Percentile	Raw	Percentile
37	0.00	0.00	0.22	0.07	0.00	0.00	0.00	0.00	0.00	0.00
38	0.00	0.00	0.29	0.16	0.00	0.00	0.00	0.00	0.00	0.00
39	0.00	0.00	0.35	0.16	0.00	0.00	0.00	0.00	0.00	0.00
40	0.01	0.29	0.42	0.16	0.00	0.29	0.00	0.00	0.02	0.30
41	0.09	0.29	0.49	0.16	0.06	0.29	0.00	0.00	0.09	0.30
42	0.16	0.29	0.56	0.24	0.13	0.29	0.00	0.00	0.17	0.30
43	0.23	0.29	0.63	0.24	0.19	0.29	0.00	0.00	0.25	0.30
44	0.31	0.43	0.70	0.25	0.25	0.29	0.04	0.57	0.32	0.42
45	0.38	0.43	0.76	0.37	0.31	0.45	0.09	0.57	0.40	0.42
46	0.45	0.43	0.83	0.37	0.37	0.45	0.15	0.57	0.47	0.42
47	0.53	0.56	0.90	0.37	0.43	0.45	0.20	0.57	0.55	0.55
48	0.60	0.56	0.97	0.37	0.49	0.45	0.26	0.69	0.62	0.55
49	0.67	0.56	1.04	0.49	0.55	0.62	0.31	0.69	0.70	0.55
50	0.75	0.56	1.11	0.49	0.61	0.62	0.37	0.69	0.77	0.65
51	0.82	0.64	1.17	0.49	0.68	0.62	0.42	0.69	0.85	0.65
52	0.90	0.64	1.24	0.49	0.74	0.62	0.48	0.69	0.92	0.65

Table A–8. Personality Inventory for DSM-5—Self-Report Form (100 item) normative tables: trait scales (continued)

T	Separation insecurity		Submissiveness		Suspiciousness		Unusual beliefs and experiences		Withdrawal	
	Raw	Percentile	Raw	Percentile	Raw	Percentile	Raw	Percentile	Raw	Percentile
53	0.97	0.64	1.31	0.60	0.80	0.75	0.53	0.79	1.00	0.75
54	1.04	0.74	1.38	0.60	0.86	0.75	0.59	0.79	1.08	0.75
55	1.12	0.74	1.45	0.60	0.92	0.75	0.64	0.79	1.15	0.75
56	1.19	0.74	1.52	0.71	0.98	0.75	0.70	0.79	1.23	0.75
57	1.26	0.81	1.58	0.71	1.04	0.85	0.75	0.86	1.30	0.81
58	1.34	0.81	1.65	0.71	1.10	0.85	0.81	0.86	1.38	0.82
59	1.41	0.81	1.72	0.72	1.17	0.85	0.86	0.86	1.45	0.82
60	1.48	0.81	1.79	0.84	1.23	0.85	0.92	0.86	1.53	0.88
61	1.56	0.87	1.86	0.84	1.29	0.90	0.97	0.86	1.60	0.88
62	1.63	0.87	1.93	0.84	1.35	0.90	1.03	0.91	1.68	0.88
63	1.71	0.87	2.00	0.84	1.41	0.90	1.08	0.91	1.75	0.94
64	1.78	0.91	2.06	0.93	1.47	0.90	1.14	0.91	1.83	0.94
65	1.85	0.91	2.13	0.93	1.53	0.94	1.19	0.91	1.91	0.94
66	1.93	0.91	2.20	0.93	1.59	0.94	1.25	0.91	1.98	0.94
67	2.00	0.91	2.27	0.98	1.65	0.94	1.30	0.95	2.06	0.97
68	2.07	0.94	2.34	0.98	1.72	0.95	1.36	0.95	2.13	0.97

Table A–8. Personality Inventory for DSM-5—Self-Report Form (100 item) normative tables: trait scales *(continued)*

T	Separation insecurity		Submissiveness		Suspiciousness		Unusual beliefs and experiences		Withdrawal	
	Raw	Percentile	Raw	Percentile	Raw	Percentile	Raw	Percentile	Raw	Percentile
69	2.15	0.94	2.41	0.98	1.78	0.98	1.41	0.95	2.21	0.97
70	2.22	0.94	2.47	0.98	1.84	0.98	1.46	0.95	2.28	0.98
71	2.29	0.97	2.54	1.00	1.90	0.98	1.52	0.97	2.36	0.98
72	2.37	0.98	2.61	1.00	1.96	0.98	1.57	0.97	2.43	0.98
73	2.44	0.98	2.68	1.00	2.02	0.99	1.63	0.97	2.51	0.99
74	2.51	0.99	2.75	1.00	2.08	0.99	1.68	0.97	2.59	0.99
75	2.59	0.99	2.82	1.00	2.14	0.99	1.74	0.97	2.66	0.99
76	2.66	0.99	2.88	1.00	2.20	0.99	1.79	0.98	2.74	0.99
77	2.74	0.99	2.95	1.00	2.27	0.99	1.85	0.98	2.81	0.99
78	2.81	1.00	3.02	1.00	2.33	0.99	1.90	0.98	2.89	0.99
79	2.88	1.00	3.09	1.00	2.39	0.99	1.96	0.98	2.96	0.99
80	2.96	1.00	3.16	1.00	2.45	0.99	2.01	0.99	3.04	1.00
81	3.03	1.00	3.23	1.00	2.51	0.99	2.07	0.99	3.11	1.00
82	3.10	1.00	3.29	1.00	2.57	0.99	2.12	0.99	3.19	1.00
83	3.18	1.00	3.36	1.00	2.63	0.99	2.18	0.99	3.26	1.00
84	3.25	1.00	3.43	1.00	2.69	1.00	2.23	0.99	3.34	1.00

Table A–8. Personality Inventory for DSM-5—Self-Report Form (100 item) normative tables: trait scales *(continued)*

T	Separation insecurity		Submissiveness		Suspiciousness		Unusual beliefs and experiences		Withdrawal	
	Raw	Percentile	Raw	Percentile	Raw	Percentile	Raw	Percentile	Raw	Percentile
85	3.32	1.00	3.50	1.00	2.76	1.00	2.29	1.00	3.42	1.00
86	3.40	1.00	3.57	1.00	2.82	1.00	2.34	1.00	3.49	1.00
87	3.47	1.00	3.64	1.00	2.88	1.00	2.40	1.00	3.57	1.00
88	3.55	1.00	3.70	1.00	2.94	1.00	2.45	1.00	3.64	1.00
89	3.62	1.00	3.77	1.00	3.00	1.00	2.51	1.00	3.72	1.00
90	3.69	1.00	3.84	1.00	3.06	1.00	2.56	1.00	3.79	1.00
91	3.77	1.00	3.91	1.00	3.12	1.00	2.62	1.00	3.87	1.00
92	3.84	1.00	3.98	1.00	3.18	1.00	2.67	1.00	3.94	1.00
93	3.91	1.00	4.00	1.00	3.24	1.00	2.73	1.00	4.00	1.00
94	3.99	1.00	4.00	1.00	3.31	1.00	2.78	1.00	4.00	1.00
95	4.00	1.00	4.00	1.00	3.37	1.00	2.84	1.00	4.00	1.00
96	4.00	1.00	4.00	1.00	3.43	1.00	2.89	1.00	4.00	1.00
97	4.00	1.00	4.00	1.00	3.49	1.00	2.94	1.00	4.00	1.00
98	4.00	1.00	4.00	1.00	3.55	1.00	3.00	1.00	4.00	1.00
99	4.00	1.00	4.00	1.00	3.61	1.00	3.05	1.00	4.00	1.00
100	4.00	1.00	4.00	1.00	3.67	1.00	3.11	1.00	4.00	1.00

Table A–9. Personality Inventory for DSM-5—Brief Form normative tables: total score and domain scales

T	Total		Negative affect		Detachment		Antagonism		Disinhibition		Psychoticism	
	Raw	Percentile	Raw	Percentile	Raw	Percentile	Raw	Percentile	Raw	Percentile	Raw	Percentile
35	0.00	0.00	0.00	0.00	0.00	0.00	0.00	0.00	0.00	0.00	0.00	0.00
36	0.00	0.00	0.00	0.00	0.00	0.00	0.00	0.00	0.00	0.00	0.00	0.00
37	0.00	0.00	0.00	0.00	0.00	0.00	0.00	0.00	0.00	0.00	0.00	0.00
38	0.01	0.04	0.00	0.00	0.00	0.00	0.00	0.00	0.00	0.00	0.00	0.00
39	0.06	0.08	0.00	0.00	0.00	0.00	0.00	0.00	0.00	0.00	0.00	0.00
40	0.10	0.12	0.06	0.21	0.04	0.24	0.00	0.00	0.00	0.00	0.00	0.00
41	0.15	0.16	0.12	0.21	0.11	0.24	0.00	0.00	0.05	0.24	0.00	0.00
42	0.19	0.22	0.19	0.21	0.17	0.24	0.00	0.40	0.10	0.24	0.00	0.00
43	0.24	0.27	0.26	0.33	0.23	0.35	0.05	0.40	0.16	0.24	0.04	0.44
44	0.28	0.34	0.32	0.33	0.30	0.36	0.10	0.40	0.22	0.41	0.09	0.44
45	0.33	0.40	0.39	0.33	0.36	0.36	0.15	0.40	0.27	0.41	0.15	0.44
46	0.37	0.44	0.46	0.47	0.42	0.47	0.20	0.40	0.33	0.41	0.21	0.55
47	0.42	0.49	0.52	0.47	0.48	0.47	0.25	0.55	0.39	0.41	0.26	0.56
48	0.47	0.52	0.59	0.47	0.55	0.47	0.30	0.56	0.44	0.57	0.32	0.56
49	0.51	0.55	0.66	0.56	0.61	0.59	0.35	0.56	0.50	0.57	0.38	0.56
50	0.56	0.59	0.72	0.56	0.67	0.59	0.40	0.56	0.56	0.58	0.44	0.68

Table A–9. Personality Inventory for DSM-5—Brief Form normative tables: total score and domain scales *(continued)*

T	Total		Negative affect		Detachment		Antagonism		Disinhibition		Psychoticism	
	Raw	Percentile	Raw	Percentile	Raw	Percentile	Raw	Percentile	Raw	Percentile	Raw	Percentile
51	0.60	0.65	0.79	0.56	0.74	0.59	0.44	0.69	0.61	0.69	0.49	0.68
52	0.65	0.66	0.86	0.66	0.80	0.59	0.49	0.69	0.67	0.70	0.55	0.68
53	0.69	0.69	0.92	0.66	0.86	0.68	0.54	0.69	0.73	0.70	0.61	0.75
54	0.74	0.71	0.99	0.66	0.92	0.68	0.59	0.69	0.78	0.70	0.66	0.75
55	0.78	0.73	1.06	0.74	0.99	0.68	0.64	0.77	0.84	0.78	0.72	0.75
56	0.83	0.75	1.12	0.74	1.05	0.77	0.69	0.77	0.89	0.78	0.78	0.75
57	0.87	0.78	1.19	0.74	1.11	0.77	0.74	0.77	0.95	0.78	0.84	0.81
58	0.92	0.82	1.25	0.81	1.18	0.77	0.79	0.78	1.01	0.84	0.89	0.81
59	0.97	0.84	1.32	0.81	1.24	0.83	0.84	0.85	1.06	0.84	0.95	0.81
60	1.01	0.85	1.39	0.81	1.30	0.83	0.89	0.85	1.12	0.84	1.01	0.86
61	1.06	0.87	1.45	0.86	1.36	0.83	0.94	0.85	1.18	0.84	1.06	0.86
62	1.10	0.87	1.52	0.86	1.43	0.88	0.99	0.85	1.23	0.89	1.12	0.86
63	1.15	0.89	1.59	0.86	1.49	0.88	1.03	0.92	1.29	0.89	1.18	0.86
64	1.19	0.90	1.65	0.90	1.55	0.88	1.08	0.92	1.35	0.89	1.23	0.90
65	1.24	0.91	1.72	0.90	1.62	0.92	1.13	0.92	1.40	0.92	1.29	0.90
66	1.28	0.93	1.79	0.90	1.68	0.92	1.18	0.92	1.46	0.92	1.35	0.91

Table A–9. Personality Inventory for DSM-5—Brief Form normative tables: total score and domain scales *(continued)*

T	Total		Negative affect		Detachment		Antagonism		Disinhibition		Psychoticism	
	Raw	Percentile	Raw	Percentile	Raw	Percentile	Raw	Percentile	Raw	Percentile	Raw	Percentile
67	1.33	0.93	1.85	0.93	1.74	0.92	1.23	0.93	1.52	0.92	1.41	0.94
68	1.37	0.94	1.92	0.93	1.81	0.96	1.28	0.93	1.57	0.92	1.46	0.94
69	1.42	0.94	1.99	0.93	1.87	0.96	1.33	0.93	1.63	0.95	1.52	0.94
70	1.47	0.95	2.05	0.95	1.93	0.96	1.38	0.93	1.69	0.95	1.58	0.94
71	1.51	0.95	2.12	0.95	1.99	0.96	1.43	0.96	1.74	0.95	1.63	0.96
72	1.56	0.95	2.19	0.95	2.06	0.98	1.48	0.96	1.80	0.95	1.69	0.96
73	1.60	0.96	2.25	0.98	2.12	0.98	1.53	0.96	1.85	0.96	1.75	0.96
74	1.65	0.97	2.32	0.98	2.18	0.98	1.57	0.96	1.91	0.96	1.81	0.97
75	1.69	0.98	2.39	0.98	2.25	0.99	1.62	0.98	1.97	0.96	1.86	0.97
76	1.74	0.98	2.45	0.98	2.31	0.99	1.67	0.98	2.02	0.98	1.92	0.97
77	1.78	0.98	2.52	0.98	2.37	0.99	1.72	0.98	2.08	0.98	1.98	0.97
78	1.83	0.99	2.59	0.98	2.43	0.99	1.77	0.98	2.14	0.98	2.03	0.98
79	1.87	0.99	2.65	0.99	2.50	0.99	1.82	0.98	2.19	0.98	2.09	0.98
80	1.92	0.99	2.72	0.99	2.56	0.99	1.87	0.98	2.25	0.99	2.15	0.98
81	1.97	0.99	2.79	0.99	2.62	0.99	1.92	0.98	2.31	0.99	2.21	0.99
82	2.01	0.99	2.85	1.00	2.69	0.99	1.97	0.98	2.36	0.99	2.26	0.99

Table A–9. Personality Inventory for DSM-5—Brief Form normative tables: total score and domain scales *(continued)*

T	Total		Negative affect		Detachment		Antagonism		Disinhibition		Psychoticism	
	Raw	Percentile	Raw	Percentile	Raw	Percentile	Raw	Percentile	Raw	Percentile	Raw	Percentile
83	2.06	0.99	2.92	1.00	2.75	0.99	2.02	0.99	2.42	0.99	2.32	0.99
84	2.10	0.99	2.98	1.00	2.81	1.00	2.07	0.99	2.48	0.99	2.38	0.99
85	2.15	1.00	3.05	1.00	2.87	1.00	2.11	0.99	2.53	0.99	2.43	1.00
86	2.19	1.00	3.12	1.00	2.94	1.00	2.16	0.99	2.59	0.99	2.49	1.00
87	2.24	1.00	3.18	1.00	3.00	1.00	2.21	0.99	2.65	1.00	2.55	1.00
88	2.28	1.00	3.25	1.00	3.06	1.00	2.26	0.99	2.70	1.00	2.61	1.00
89	2.33	1.00	3.32	1.00	3.13	1.00	2.31	0.99	2.76	1.00	2.66	1.00
90	2.37	1.00	3.38	1.00	3.19	1.00	2.36	0.99	2.81	1.00	2.72	1.00
91	2.42	1.00	3.45	1.00	3.25	1.00	2.41	1.00	2.87	1.00	2.78	1.00
92	2.47	1.00	3.52	1.00	3.31	1.00	2.46	1.00	2.93	1.00	2.83	1.00
93	2.51	1.00	3.58	1.00	3.38	1.00	2.51	1.00	2.98	1.00	2.89	1.00
94	2.56	1.00	3.65	1.00	3.44	1.00	2.56	1.00	3.04	1.00	2.95	1.00
95	2.60	1.00	3.72	1.00	3.50	1.00	2.61	1.00	3.10	1.00	3.00	1.00

Table A–10.   Personality Inventory for DSM-5—Informant Form normative tables: domain scales

T	Negative affect		Detachment		Antagonism		Disinhibition		Psychoticism	
	Raw	Percentile	Raw	Percentile	Raw	Percentile	Raw	Percentile	Raw	Percentile
35	0.00	0.00	0.00	0.00	0.00	0.00	0.00	0.00	0.00	0.00
36	0.00	0.00	0.00	0.00	0.00	0.00	0.00	0.00	0.00	0.00
37	0.00	0.00	0.02	0.02	0.00	0.00	0.00	0.00	0.00	0.00
38	0.04	0.04	0.08	0.07	0.00	0.00	0.00	0.00	0.00	0.00
39	0.10	0.11	0.13	0.11	0.00	0.00	0.02	0.08	0.00	0.00
40	0.17	0.18	0.19	0.15	0.06	0.09	0.08	0.15	0.00	0.00
41	0.23	0.22	0.25	0.21	0.12	0.15	0.14	0.21	0.00	0.00
42	0.29	0.27	0.31	0.26	0.19	0.22	0.20	0.25	0.04	0.21
43	0.36	0.33	0.37	0.32	0.25	0.28	0.26	0.31	0.08	0.34
44	0.42	0.37	0.42	0.35	0.32	0.36	0.31	0.36	0.13	0.39
45	0.49	0.40	0.48	0.38	0.38	0.42	0.37	0.42	0.18	0.45
46	0.55	0.43	0.54	0.43	0.45	0.47	0.43	0.45	0.23	0.50
47	0.61	0.47	0.60	0.47	0.51	0.52	0.49	0.49	0.27	0.54
48	0.68	0.50	0.66	0.51	0.57	0.54	0.55	0.52	0.32	0.57
49	0.74	0.53	0.71	0.54	0.64	0.57	0.61	0.55	0.37	0.60
50	0.81	0.57	0.77	0.57	0.70	0.60	0.66	0.61	0.41	0.62

Table A–10. Personality Inventory for DSM-5—Informant Form normative tables: domain scales *(continued)*

T	Negative affect		Detachment		Antagonism		Disinhibition		Psychoticism	
	Raw	Percentile	Raw	Percentile	Raw	Percentile	Raw	Percentile	Raw	Percentile
51	0.87	0.59	0.83	0.60	0.77	0.63	0.72	0.64	0.46	0.65
52	0.93	0.63	0.89	0.64	0.83	0.67	0.78	0.64	0.51	0.66
53	1.00	0.66	0.95	0.65	0.90	0.69	0.84	0.66	0.56	0.70
54	1.06	0.69	1.00	0.69	0.96	0.72	0.90	0.68	0.60	0.72
55	1.13	0.70	1.06	0.70	1.02	0.73	0.96	0.72	0.65	0.76
56	1.19	0.73	1.12	0.73	1.09	0.77	1.01	0.73	0.70	0.78
57	1.25	0.75	1.18	0.76	1.15	0.79	1.07	0.76	0.74	0.79
58	1.32	0.77	1.24	0.79	1.22	0.82	1.13	0.78	0.79	0.81
59	1.38	0.80	1.29	0.80	1.28	0.84	1.19	0.80	0.84	0.84
60	1.44	0.82	1.35	0.83	1.35	0.84	1.25	0.83	0.89	0.85
61	1.51	0.84	1.41	0.85	1.41	0.85	1.31	0.85	0.93	0.86
62	1.57	0.87	1.47	0.87	1.47	0.86	1.36	0.86	0.98	0.87
63	1.64	0.88	1.53	0.89	1.54	0.87	1.42	0.87	1.03	0.89
64	1.70	0.90	1.58	0.90	1.60	0.88	1.48	0.89	1.08	0.91
65	1.76	0.91	1.64	0.91	1.67	0.90	1.54	0.91	1.12	0.92
66	1.83	0.92	1.70	0.92	1.73	0.91	1.60	0.92	1.17	0.93

Table A–10.   Personality Inventory for DSM-5 – Informant Form normative tables: domain scales *(continued)*

T	Negative affect		Detachment		Antagonism		Disinhibition		Psychoticism	
	Raw	Percentile	Raw	Percentile	Raw	Percentile	Raw	Percentile	Raw	Percentile
67	1.89	0.92	1.76	0.93	1.80	0.92	1.66	0.93	1.22	0.93
68	1.96	0.94	1.82	0.93	1.86	0.94	1.71	0.94	1.26	0.93
69	2.02	0.94	1.87	0.94	1.93	0.94	1.77	0.95	1.31	0.94
70	2.08	0.96	1.93	0.94	1.99	0.96	1.83	0.96	1.36	0.95
71	2.15	0.96	1.99	0.96	2.05	0.96	1.89	0.96	1.41	0.95
72	2.21	0.97	2.05	0.97	2.12	0.96	1.95	0.97	1.45	0.96
73	2.28	0.98	2.11	0.97	2.18	0.97	2.01	0.98	1.50	0.96
74	2.34	0.98	2.16	0.98	2.25	0.97	2.06	0.98	1.55	0.96
75	2.40	0.99	2.22	0.99	2.31	0.97	2.12	0.98	1.59	0.97
76	2.47	0.99	2.28	0.99	2.38	0.97	2.18	0.99	1.64	0.97
77	2.53	0.99	2.34	0.99	2.44	0.97	2.24	0.99	1.69	0.98
78	2.60	0.99	2.40	0.99	2.50	0.98	2.30	0.99	1.74	0.98
79	2.66	0.99	2.45	0.99	2.57	0.98	2.36	0.99	1.78	0.98
80	2.72	1.00	2.51	1.00	2.63	0.98	2.41	0.99	1.83	0.98
81	2.79	1.00	2.57	1.00	2.70	0.98	2.47	0.99	1.88	0.99
82	2.85	1.00	2.63	1.00	2.76	0.99	2.53	0.99	1.93	0.99

Table A–10. Personality Inventory for DSM-5—Informant Form normative tables: domain scales *(continued)*

T	Negative affect		Detachment		Antagonism		Disinhibition		Psychoticism	
	Raw	Percentile	Raw	Percentile	Raw	Percentile	Raw	Percentile	Raw	Percentile
83	2.91	1.00	2.69	1.00	2.83	1.00	2.59	0.99	1.97	0.99
84	2.98	1.00	2.74	1.00	2.89	1.00	2.65	0.99	2.02	0.99
85	3.04	1.00	2.80	1.00	2.95	1.00	2.71	1.00	2.07	0.99
86	3.11	1.00	2.86	1.00	3.02	1.00	2.76	1.00	2.11	0.99
87	3.17	1.00	2.92	1.00	3.08	1.00	2.82	1.00	2.16	0.99
88	3.23	1.00	2.98	1.00	3.15	1.00	2.88	1.00	2.21	0.99
89	3.30	1.00	3.03	1.00	3.21	1.00	2.94	1.00	2.26	1.00
90	3.36	1.00	3.09	1.00	3.28	1.00	3.00	1.00	2.30	1.00

Table A–11. Personality Inventory for DSM-5 — Informant Form normative tables: trait scales

T	Anhedonia		Anxiousness		Attention seeking		Callousness		Deceitfulness	
	Raw	Percentile	Raw	Percentile	Raw	Percentile	Raw	Percentile	Raw	Percentile
30	0.00	0.00	0.00	0.00	0.00	0.00	0.00	0.00	0.00	0.00
31	0.00	0.00	0.00	0.00	0.00	0.00	0.00	0.00	0.00	0.00
32	0.00	0.00	0.00	0.00	0.00	0.00	0.00	0.00	0.00	0.00
33	0.00	0.00	0.00	0.00	0.00	0.00	0.00	0.00	0.00	0.00
34	0.00	0.00	0.00	0.00	0.00	0.00	0.00	0.00	0.00	0.00
35	0.00	0.00	0.00	0.00	0.00	0.00	0.00	0.00	0.00	0.00
36	0.00	0.00	0.00	0.00	0.00	0.00	0.00	0.00	0.00	0.00
37	0.00	0.00	0.00	0.00	0.00	0.00	0.00	0.00	0.00	0.00
38	0.00	0.00	0.00	0.00	0.00	0.00	0.00	0.00	0.00	0.00
39	0.06	0.10	0.00	0.00	0.00	0.00	0.00	0.00	0.00	0.00
40	0.13	0.17	0.06	0.22	0.07	0.18	0.00	0.00	0.00	0.00
41	0.20	0.18	0.14	0.28	0.15	0.25	0.00	0.00	0.00	0.00
42	0.27	0.29	0.21	0.28	0.23	0.26	0.03	0.28	0.03	0.28
43	0.34	0.29	0.29	0.36	0.32	0.35	0.09	0.36	0.09	0.36
44	0.40	0.36	0.37	0.36	0.40	0.41	0.15	0.44	0.15	0.44
45	0.47	0.36	0.44	0.43	0.48	0.41	0.22	0.49	0.22	0.49

Table A–11. Personality Inventory for DSM-5—Informant Form normative tables: trait scales *(continued)*

T	Anhedonia		Anxiousness		Attention seeking		Callousness		Deceitfulness	
	Raw	Percentile	Raw	Percentile	Raw	Percentile	Raw	Percentile	Raw	Percentile
46	0.54	0.44	0.52	0.47	0.56	0.47	0.28	0.50	0.28	0.50
47	0.61	0.44	0.60	0.47	0.64	0.51	0.34	0.54	0.34	0.54
48	0.68	0.52	0.67	0.49	0.72	0.52	0.41	0.57	0.41	0.57
49	0.75	0.53	0.75	0.49	0.81	0.55	0.47	0.60	0.47	0.60
50	0.81	0.60	0.83	0.54	0.89	0.59	0.53	0.63	0.53	0.63
51	0.88	0.66	0.90	0.58	0.97	0.59	0.60	0.66	0.60	0.66
52	0.95	0.66	0.98	0.58	1.05	0.61	0.66	0.67	0.66	0.67
53	1.02	0.70	1.06	0.65	1.13	0.64	0.72	0.71	0.72	0.71
54	1.09	0.70	1.13	0.71	1.21	0.65	0.79	0.74	0.79	0.74
55	1.16	0.73	1.21	0.71	1.30	0.70	0.85	0.74	0.85	0.74
56	1.22	0.73	1.29	0.74	1.38	0.74	0.92	0.75	0.92	0.75
57	1.29	0.79	1.36	0.74	1.46	0.74	0.98	0.77	0.98	0.77
58	1.36	0.79	1.44	0.78	1.54	0.78	1.04	0.79	1.04	0.79
59	1.43	0.82	1.52	0.81	1.62	0.78	1.11	0.82	1.11	0.82
60	1.50	0.82	1.59	0.81	1.70	0.82	1.17	0.84	1.17	0.84
61	1.57	0.86	1.67	0.85	1.79	0.84	1.23	0.85	1.23	0.85

Table A–11. Personality Inventory for DSM-5—Informant Form normative tables: trait scales (continued)

T	Anhedonia		Anxiousness		Attention seeking		Callousness		Deceitfulness	
	Raw	Percentile	Raw	Percentile	Raw	Percentile	Raw	Percentile	Raw	Percentile
62	1.63	0.88	1.75	0.85	1.87	0.85	1.30	0.86	1.30	0.86
63	1.70	0.88	1.82	0.87	1.95	0.88	1.36	0.87	1.36	0.87
64	1.77	0.90	1.90	0.89	2.03	0.90	1.42	0.88	1.42	0.88
65	1.84	0.90	1.98	0.89	2.11	0.90	1.49	0.89	1.49	0.89
66	1.91	0.91	2.05	0.92	2.19	0.91	1.55	0.90	1.55	0.90
67	1.98	0.91	2.13	0.93	2.28	0.92	1.61	0.92	1.61	0.92
68	2.05	0.92	2.21	0.93	2.36	0.92	1.68	0.93	1.68	0.93
69	2.11	0.92	2.28	0.96	2.44	0.94	1.74	0.94	1.74	0.94
70	2.18	0.95	2.36	0.96	2.52	0.95	1.80	0.95	1.80	0.95
71	2.25	0.96	2.43	0.97	2.60	0.95	1.87	0.95	1.87	0.95
72	2.32	0.96	2.51	0.97	2.68	0.96	1.93	0.96	1.93	0.96
73	2.39	0.97	2.59	0.97	2.77	0.98	1.99	0.96	1.99	0.96
74	2.46	0.97	2.66	0.99	2.85	0.98	2.06	0.97	2.06	0.97
75	2.52	0.98	2.74	0.99	2.93	0.99	2.12	0.97	2.12	0.97
76	2.59	0.98	2.82	0.99	3.01	1.00	2.19	0.97	2.19	0.97
77	2.66	0.98	2.89	0.99	3.09	1.00	2.25	0.97	2.25	0.97

Table A–11. Personality Inventory for DSM-5—Informant Form normative tables: trait scales *(continued)*

T	Anhedonia		Anxiousness		Attention seeking		Callousness		Deceitfulness	
	Raw	Percentile	Raw	Percentile	Raw	Percentile	Raw	Percentile	Raw	Percentile
78	2.73	0.98	2.97	0.99	3.17	1.00	2.31	0.98	2.31	0.98
79	2.80	0.99	3.05	1.00	3.26	1.00	2.38	0.98	2.38	0.98
80	2.87	0.99	3.12	1.00	3.34	1.00	2.44	0.99	2.44	0.99
81	2.93	0.99	3.20	1.00	3.42	1.00	2.50	0.99	2.50	0.99
82	3.00	1.00	3.28	1.00	3.50	1.00	2.57	0.99	2.57	0.99
83	3.07	1.00	3.35	1.00	3.58	1.00	2.63	0.99	2.63	0.99
84	3.14	1.00	3.43	1.00	3.67	1.00	2.69	1.00	2.69	1.00
85	3.21	1.00	3.51	1.00	3.75	1.00	2.76	1.00	2.76	1.00
86	3.28	1.00	3.58	1.00	3.83	1.00	2.82	1.00	2.82	1.00
87	3.34	1.00	3.66	1.00	3.91	1.00	2.88	1.00	2.88	1.00
88	3.41	1.00	3.74	1.00	3.99	1.00	2.95	1.00	2.95	1.00
89	3.48	1.00	3.81	1.00	4.00	1.00	3.01	1.00	3.01	1.00
90	3.55	1.00	3.89	1.00	4.00	1.00	3.07	1.00	3.07	1.00
91	3.62	1.00	3.97	1.00	4.00	1.00	3.14	1.00	3.14	1.00
92	3.69	1.00	4.00	1.00	4.00	1.00	3.20	1.00	3.20	1.00
93	3.75	1.00	4.00	1.00	4.00	1.00	3.26	1.00	3.26	1.00
94	3.82	1.00	4.00	1.00	4.00	1.00	3.33	1.00	3.33	1.00

Table A–11. Personality Inventory for DSM-5–Informant Form normative tables: trait scales (continued)

T	Anhedonia		Anxiousness		Attention seeking		Callousness		Deceitfulness	
	Raw	Percentile	Raw	Percentile	Raw	Percentile	Raw	Percentile	Raw	Percentile
95	3.89	1.00	4.00	1.00	4.00	1.00	3.39	1.00	3.39	1.00
96	3.96	1.00	4.00	1.00	4.00	1.00	3.45	1.00	3.45	1.00
97	4.00	1.00	4.00	1.00	4.00	1.00	3.52	1.00	3.52	1.00
98	4.00	1.00	4.00	1.00	4.00	1.00	3.58	1.00	3.58	1.00
99	4.00	1.00	4.00	1.00	4.00	1.00	3.65	1.00	3.65	1.00
100	4.00	1.00	4.00	1.00	4.00	1.00	3.71	1.00	3.71	1.00
101	4.00	1.00	4.00	1.00	4.00	1.00	3.77	1.00	3.77	1.00
102	4.00	1.00	4.00	1.00	4.00	1.00	3.84	1.00	3.84	1.00
103	4.00	1.00	4.00	1.00	4.00	1.00	3.90	1.00	3.90	1.00
104	4.00	1.00	4.00	1.00	4.00	1.00	3.96	1.00	3.96	1.00
105	4.00	1.00	4.00	1.00	4.00	1.00	4.00	1.00	4.00	1.00
106	4.00	1.00	4.00	1.00	4.00	1.00	4.00	1.00	4.00	1.00
107	4.00	1.00	4.00	1.00	4.00	1.00	4.00	1.00	4.00	1.00
108	4.00	1.00	4.00	1.00	4.00	1.00	4.00	1.00	4.00	1.00
109	4.00	1.00	4.00	1.00	4.00	1.00	4.00	1.00	4.00	1.00
110	4.00	1.00	4.00	1.00	4.00	1.00	4.00	1.00	4.00	1.00

Table A-11. Personality Inventory for DSM-5—Informant Form normative tables: trait scales *(continued)*

T	Depressivity		Distractibility		Eccentricity		Emotional lability		Grandiosity	
	Raw	Percentile	Raw	Percentile	Raw	Percentile	Raw	Percentile	Raw	Percentile
30	0.00	0.00	0.00	0.00	0.00	0.00	0.00	0.00	0.00	0.00
31	0.00	0.00	0.00	0.00	0.00	0.00	0.00	0.00	0.00	0.00
32	0.00	0.00	0.00	0.00	0.00	0.00	0.00	0.00	0.00	0.00
33	0.00	0.00	0.00	0.00	0.00	0.00	0.00	0.00	0.00	0.00
34	0.00	0.00	0.00	0.00	0.00	0.00	0.00	0.00	0.00	0.00
35	0.00	0.00	0.00	0.00	0.00	0.00	0.00	0.00	0.00	0.00
36	0.00	0.00	0.00	0.00	0.00	0.00	0.00	0.00	0.00	0.00
37	0.00	0.00	0.00	0.00	0.00	0.00	0.00	0.00	0.00	0.00
38	0.00	0.00	0.00	0.00	0.00	0.00	0.00	0.00	0.00	0.00
39	0.00	0.00	0.00	0.00	0.00	0.00	0.00	0.00	0.00	0.00
40	0.00	0.00	0.04	0.21	0.00	0.00	0.06	0.17	0.00	0.00
41	0.00	0.00	0.10	0.21	0.02	0.21	0.14	0.17	0.00	0.00
42	0.03	0.25	0.17	0.29	0.09	0.29	0.22	0.29	0.03	0.36
43	0.09	0.35	0.24	0.37	0.16	0.38	0.29	0.36	0.11	0.36
44	0.15	0.42	0.31	0.38	0.23	0.44	0.37	0.36	0.19	0.47
45	0.21	0.42	0.38	0.45	0.30	0.44	0.45	0.45	0.27	0.48

Table A–11. Personality Inventory for DSM-5—Informant Form normative tables: trait scales *(continued)*

T	Depressivity Raw	Percentile	Distractibility Raw	Percentile	Eccentricity Raw	Percentile	Emotional lability Raw	Percentile	Grandiosity Raw	Percentile
46	0.27	0.46	0.44	0.49	0.37	0.49	0.52	0.46	0.35	0.53
47	0.34	0.54	0.51	0.50	0.44	0.53	0.60	0.51	0.43	0.54
48	0.40	0.58	0.58	0.54	0.51	0.56	0.67	0.52	0.51	0.58
49	0.46	0.62	0.65	0.54	0.58	0.59	0.75	0.57	0.59	0.58
50	0.52	0.65	0.72	0.56	0.65	0.61	0.83	0.57	0.66	0.59
51	0.58	0.68	0.79	0.60	0.72	0.63	0.90	0.61	0.74	0.64
52	0.64	0.68	0.85	0.60	0.79	0.65	0.98	0.61	0.82	0.64
53	0.70	0.70	0.92	0.65	0.86	0.67	1.06	0.67	0.90	0.70
54	0.77	0.73	0.99	0.65	0.93	0.69	1.13	0.67	0.98	0.70
55	0.83	0.76	1.06	0.69	1.01	0.72	1.21	0.71	1.06	0.73
56	0.89	0.78	1.13	0.73	1.08	0.72	1.29	0.71	1.14	0.73
57	0.95	0.80	1.20	0.73	1.15	0.73	1.36	0.76	1.22	0.78
58	1.01	0.82	1.26	0.77	1.22	0.77	1.44	0.79	1.30	0.78
59	1.07	0.83	1.33	0.77	1.29	0.80	1.51	0.79	1.38	0.81
60	1.13	0.83	1.40	0.81	1.36	0.83	1.59	0.83	1.46	0.82
61	1.20	0.84	1.47	0.84	1.43	0.86	1.67	0.84	1.54	0.85

Table A–11. Personality Inventory for DSM-5—Informant Form normative tables: trait scales (continued)

T	Depressivity		Distractibility		Eccentricity		Emotional lability		Grandiosity	
	Raw	Percentile	Raw	Percentile	Raw	Percentile	Raw	Percentile	Raw	Percentile
62	1.26	0.85	1.54	0.85	1.50	0.87	1.74	0.86	1.62	0.85
63	1.32	0.88	1.61	0.89	1.57	0.88	1.82	0.86	1.70	0.86
64	1.38	0.89	1.67	0.91	1.64	0.89	1.90	0.89	1.78	0.86
65	1.44	0.90	1.74	0.91	1.71	0.90	1.97	0.89	1.85	0.90
66	1.50	0.91	1.81	0.93	1.78	0.91	2.05	0.91	1.93	0.90
67	1.56	0.91	1.88	0.93	1.85	0.92	2.13	0.91	2.01	0.95
68	1.63	0.92	1.95	0.95	1.92	0.92	2.20	0.95	2.09	0.95
69	1.69	0.92	2.01	0.96	1.99	0.94	2.28	0.95	2.17	0.95
70	1.75	0.93	2.08	0.96	2.06	0.96	2.35	0.96	2.25	0.95
71	1.81	0.95	2.15	0.98	2.13	0.96	2.43	0.97	2.33	0.95
72	1.87	0.95	2.22	0.98	2.20	0.97	2.51	0.97	2.41	0.96
73	1.93	0.96	2.29	0.98	2.27	0.97	2.58	0.98	2.49	0.96
74	1.99	0.96	2.36	0.98	2.34	0.97	2.66	0.98	2.57	0.96
75	2.06	0.97	2.42	0.98	2.41	0.98	2.74	0.98	2.65	0.96
76	2.12	0.98	2.49	0.98	2.48	0.98	2.81	0.98	2.73	0.97
77	2.18	0.98	2.56	0.99	2.55	0.98	2.89	0.99	2.81	0.97

Table A-11.   Personality Inventory for DSM-5—Informant Form normative tables: trait scales (continued)

T	Depressivity		Distractibility		Eccentricity		Emotional lability		Grandiosity	
	Raw	Percentile	Raw	Percentile	Raw	Percentile	Raw	Percentile	Raw	Percentile
78	2.24	0.99	2.63	0.99	2.62	0.98	2.97	0.99	2.89	0.98
79	2.30	0.99	2.70	0.99	2.69	0.98	3.04	1.00	2.97	0.98
80	2.36	0.99	2.77	0.99	2.76	0.99	3.12	1.00	3.04	1.00
81	2.42	0.99	2.83	0.99	2.83	0.99	3.19	1.00	3.12	1.00
82	2.49	0.99	2.90	0.99	2.90	0.99	3.27	1.00	3.20	1.00
83	2.55	0.99	2.97	0.99	2.97	1.00	3.35	1.00	3.28	1.00
84	2.61	0.99	3.04	1.00	3.04	1.00	3.42	1.00	3.36	1.00
85	2.67	0.99	3.11	1.00	3.11	1.00	3.50	1.00	3.44	1.00
86	2.73	0.99	3.18	1.00	3.18	1.00	3.58	1.00	3.52	1.00
87	2.79	0.99	3.24	1.00	3.25	1.00	3.65	1.00	3.60	1.00
88	2.85	0.99	3.31	1.00	3.32	1.00	3.73	1.00	3.68	1.00
89	2.92	1.00	3.38	1.00	3.39	1.00	3.81	1.00	3.76	1.00
90	2.98	1.00	3.45	1.00	3.46	1.00	3.88	1.00	3.84	1.00
91	3.04	1.00	3.52	1.00	3.53	1.00	3.96	1.00	3.92	1.00
92	3.10	1.00	3.58	1.00	3.60	1.00	4.00	1.00	4.00	1.00
93	3.16	1.00	3.65	1.00	3.67	1.00	4.00	1.00	4.00	1.00

Table A–11. Personality Inventory for DSM-5—Informant Form normative tables: trait scales *(continued)*

T	Depressivity		Distractibility		Eccentricity		Emotional lability		Grandiosity	
	Raw	Percentile	Raw	Percentile	Raw	Percentile	Raw	Percentile	Raw	Percentile
94	3.22	1.00	3.72	1.00	3.74	1.00	4.00	1.00	4.00	1.00
95	3.28	1.00	3.79	1.00	3.81	1.00	4.00	1.00	4.00	1.00
96	3.35	1.00	3.86	1.00	3.88	1.00	4.00	1.00	4.00	1.00
97	3.41	1.00	3.93	1.00	3.95	1.00	4.00	1.00	4.00	1.00
98	3.47	1.00	3.99	1.00	4.00	1.00	4.00	1.00	4.00	1.00
99	3.53	1.00	4.00	1.00	4.00	1.00	4.00	1.00	4.00	1.00
100	3.59	1.00	4.00	1.00	4.00	1.00	4.00	1.00	4.00	1.00
101	3.65	1.00	4.00	1.00	4.00	1.00	4.00	1.00	4.00	1.00
102	3.71	1.00	4.00	1.00	4.00	1.00	4.00	1.00	4.00	1.00
103	3.78	1.00	4.00	1.00	4.00	1.00	4.00	1.00	4.00	1.00
104	3.84	1.00	4.00	1.00	4.00	1.00	4.00	1.00	4.00	1.00
105	3.90	1.00	4.00	1.00	4.00	1.00	4.00	1.00	4.00	1.00
106	3.96	1.00	4.00	1.00	4.00	1.00	4.00	1.00	4.00	1.00
107	4.00	1.00	4.00	1.00	4.00	1.00	4.00	1.00	4.00	1.00
108	4.00	1.00	4.00	1.00	4.00	1.00	4.00	1.00	4.00	1.00
109	4.00	1.00	4.00	1.00	4.00	1.00	4.00	1.00	4.00	1.00
110	4.00	1.00	4.00	1.00	4.00	1.00	4.00	1.00	4.00	1.00

Table A–11. Personality Inventory for DSM-5—Informant Form normative tables: trait scales (continued)

T	Hostility		Impulsivity		Intimacy avoidance		Irresponsibility		Manipulativeness	
	Raw	Percentile	Raw	Percentile	Raw	Percentile	Raw	Percentile	Raw	Percentile
30	0.00	0.00	0.00	0.00	0.00	0.00	0.00	0.00	0.00	0.00
31	0.00	0.00	0.00	0.00	0.00	0.00	0.00	0.00	0.00	0.00
32	0.00	0.00	0.00	0.00	0.00	0.00	0.00	0.00	0.00	0.00
33	0.00	0.00	0.00	0.00	0.00	0.00	0.00	0.00	0.00	0.00
34	0.00	0.00	0.00	0.00	0.00	0.00	0.00	0.00	0.00	0.00
35	0.00	0.00	0.00	0.00	0.00	0.00	0.00	0.00	0.00	0.00
36	0.00	0.00	0.00	0.00	0.00	0.00	0.00	0.00	0.00	0.00
37	0.00	0.00	0.00	0.00	0.00	0.00	0.00	0.00	0.00	0.00
38	0.00	0.00	0.00	0.00	0.00	0.00	0.00	0.00	0.00	0.00
39	0.03	0.13	0.03	0.18	0.00	0.00	0.00	0.00	0.05	0.13
40	0.11	0.21	0.10	0.18	0.00	0.00	0.00	0.00	0.13	0.13
41	0.19	0.22	0.18	0.27	0.02	0.27	0.00	0.00	0.20	0.13
42	0.27	0.28	0.25	0.28	0.09	0.27	0.00	0.00	0.27	0.22
43	0.35	0.33	0.32	0.28	0.17	0.27	0.05	0.37	0.34	0.22
44	0.42	0.37	0.39	0.35	0.24	0.40	0.10	0.37	0.41	0.36
45	0.50	0.42	0.46	0.36	0.31	0.40	0.16	0.51	0.56	0.36

Table A–11. Personality Inventory for DSM-5—Informant Form normative tables: trait scales *(continued)*

T	Hostility		Impulsivity		Intimacy avoidance		Irresponsibility		Manipulativeness	
	Raw	Percentile	Raw	Percentile	Raw	Percentile	Raw	Percentile	Raw	Percentile
46	0.58	0.43	0.54	0.45	0.39	0.49	0.22	0.52	0.63	0.45
47	0.66	0.47	0.61	0.46	0.46	0.50	0.28	0.52	0.70	0.45
48	0.74	0.51	0.68	0.54	0.53	0.57	0.34	0.60	0.77	0.45
49	0.81	0.56	0.75	0.54	0.61	0.58	0.39	0.60	0.85	0.55
50	0.89	0.56	0.82	0.55	0.68	0.64	0.45	0.68	0.92	0.55
51	0.97	0.59	0.89	0.61	0.75	0.65	0.51	0.68	0.99	0.55
52	1.05	0.63	0.97	0.61	0.83	0.65	0.57	0.68	1.06	0.64
53	1.13	0.66	1.04	0.69	0.90	0.69	0.63	0.72	1.14	0.64
54	1.20	0.69	1.11	0.69	0.97	0.69	0.68	0.72	1.21	0.72
55	1.28	0.69	1.18	0.73	1.05	0.74	0.74	0.75	1.28	0.72
56	1.36	0.72	1.25	0.73	1.12	0.74	0.80	0.76	1.35	0.72
57	1.44	0.76	1.33	0.73	1.19	0.78	0.86	0.81	1.42	0.79
58	1.52	0.78	1.40	0.79	1.27	0.79	0.92	0.81	1.50	0.79
59	1.60	0.78	1.47	0.79	1.34	0.82	0.97	0.81	1.57	0.79
60	1.67	0.82	1.54	0.83	1.41	0.83	1.03	0.86	1.64	0.85
61	1.75	0.84	1.61	0.83	1.49	0.83	1.09	0.86	1.71	0.85

Table A–11. Personality Inventory for DSM-5—Informant Form normative tables: trait scales (continued)

T	Hostility		Impulsivity		Intimacy avoidance		Irresponsibility		Manipulativeness	
	Raw	Percentile	Raw	Percentile	Raw	Percentile	Raw	Percentile	Raw	Percentile
62	1.83	0.87	1.69	0.88	1.56	0.86	1.15	0.89	1.78	0.85
63	1.91	0.89	1.76	0.88	1.63	0.86	1.21	0.89	1.86	0.89
64	1.99	0.89	1.83	0.88	1.71	0.89	1.27	0.89	1.93	0.89
65	2.06	0.91	1.90	0.91	1.78	0.89	1.32	0.90	2.00	0.94
66	2.14	0.93	1.97	0.91	1.85	0.92	1.38	0.91	2.07	0.94
67	2.22	0.94	2.05	0.93	1.93	0.92	1.44	0.92	2.15	0.94
68	2.30	0.94	2.12	0.93	2.00	0.95	1.50	0.92	2.22	0.95
69	2.38	0.95	2.19	0.95	2.07	0.95	1.56	0.92	2.29	0.95
70	2.45	0.95	2.26	0.95	2.15	0.95	1.61	0.94	2.36	0.95
71	2.53	0.96	2.33	0.95	2.22	0.96	1.67	0.94	2.43	0.96
72	2.61	0.97	2.40	0.97	2.29	0.96	1.73	0.96	2.51	0.96
73	2.69	0.97	2.48	0.97	2.37	0.96	1.79	0.96	2.58	0.96
74	2.77	0.97	2.55	0.98	2.44	0.96	1.85	0.96	2.65	0.98
75	2.84	0.97	2.62	0.98	2.51	0.97	1.90	0.98	2.72	0.98
76	2.92	0.99	2.69	0.99	2.59	0.97	1.96	0.98	2.79	0.98
77	3.00	1.00	2.76	0.99	2.66	0.97	2.02	0.98	2.87	0.99

Table A–11. Personality Inventory for DSM-5 — Informant Form normative tables: trait scales *(continued)*

T	Hostility		Impulsivity		Intimacy avoidance		Irresponsibility		Manipulativeness	
	Raw	Percentile	Raw	Percentile	Raw	Percentile	Raw	Percentile	Raw	Percentile
78	3.08	1.00	2.84	1.00	2.73	0.99	2.08	0.98	2.94	0.99
79	3.16	1.00	2.91	1.00	2.81	0.99	2.14	0.98	3.01	1.00
80	3.24	1.00	2.98	1.00	2.88	0.99	2.19	0.98	3.08	1.00
81	3.31	1.00	3.05	1.00	2.95	0.99	2.25	0.98	3.16	1.00
82	3.39	1.00	3.12	1.00	3.03	1.00	2.31	0.99	3.23	1.00
83	3.47	1.00	3.20	1.00	3.10	1.00	2.37	0.99	3.30	1.00
84	3.55	1.00	3.27	1.00	3.17	1.00	2.43	0.99	3.37	1.00
85	3.63	1.00	3.34	1.00	3.25	1.00	2.48	0.99	3.44	1.00
86	3.70	1.00	3.41	1.00	3.32	1.00	2.54	0.99	3.52	1.00
87	3.78	1.00	3.48	1.00	3.39	1.00	2.60	1.00	3.59	1.00
88	3.86	1.00	3.56	1.00	3.47	1.00	2.66	1.00	3.66	1.00
89	3.94	1.00	3.63	1.00	3.54	1.00	2.72	1.00	3.73	1.00
90	4.00	1.00	3.70	1.00	3.61	1.00	2.78	1.00	3.80	1.00
91	4.00	1.00	3.77	1.00	3.69	1.00	2.83	1.00	3.88	1.00
92	4.00	1.00	3.84	1.00	3.76	1.00	2.89	1.00	3.95	1.00
93	4.00	1.00	3.91	1.00	3.83	1.00	2.95	1.00	4.00	1.00

Table A–11. Personality Inventory for DSM-5 — Informant Form normative tables: trait scales *(continued)*

T	Hostility		Impulsivity		Intimacy avoidance		Irresponsibility		Manipulativeness	
	Raw	Percentile	Raw	Percentile	Raw	Percentile	Raw	Percentile	Raw	Percentile
94	4.00	1.00	3.99	1.00	3.91	1.00	3.01	1.00	4.00	1.00
95	4.00	1.00	4.00	1.00	3.98	1.00	3.07	1.00	4.00	1.00
96	4.00	1.00	4.00	1.00	4.00	1.00	3.12	1.00	4.00	1.00
97	4.00	1.00	4.00	1.00	4.00	1.00	3.18	1.00	4.00	1.00
98	4.00	1.00	4.00	1.00	4.00	1.00	3.24	1.00	4.00	1.00
99	4.00	1.00	4.00	1.00	4.00	1.00	3.30	1.00	4.00	1.00
100	4.00	1.00	4.00	1.00	4.00	1.00	3.36	1.00	4.00	1.00
101	4.00	1.00	4.00	1.00	4.00	1.00	3.41	1.00	4.00	1.00
102	4.00	1.00	4.00	1.00	4.00	1.00	3.47	1.00	4.00	1.00
103	4.00	1.00	4.00	1.00	4.00	1.00	3.53	1.00	4.00	1.00
104	4.00	1.00	4.00	1.00	4.00	1.00	3.59	1.00	4.00	1.00
105	4.00	1.00	4.00	1.00	4.00	1.00	3.65	1.00	4.00	1.00
106	4.00	1.00	4.00	1.00	4.00	1.00	3.70	1.00	4.00	1.00
107	4.00	1.00	4.00	1.00	4.00	1.00	3.76	1.00	4.00	1.00
108	4.00	1.00	4.00	1.00	4.00	1.00	3.82	1.00	4.00	1.00
109	4.00	1.00	4.00	1.00	4.00	1.00	3.88	1.00	4.00	1.00
110	4.00	1.00	4.00	1.00	4.00	1.00	3.94	1.00	4.00	1.00

Table A–11. Personality Inventory for DSM-5—Informant Form normative tables: trait scales *(continued)*

T	Perceptual dysregulation		Perseveration		Restricted affectivity		Rigid perfectionism		Risk taking	
	Raw	Percentile	Raw	Percentile	Raw	Percentile	Raw	Percentile	Raw	Percentile
30	0.00	0.00	0.00	0.00	0.00	0.00	0.00	0.00	0.00	0.00
31	0.00	0.00	0.00	0.00	0.00	0.00	0.00	0.00	0.05	0.02
32	0.00	0.00	0.00	0.00	0.00	0.00	0.00	0.00	0.10	0.04
33	0.00	0.00	0.00	0.00	0.00	0.00	0.00	0.00	0.16	0.05
34	0.00	0.00	0.00	0.00	0.00	0.00	0.00	0.00	0.22	0.06
35	0.00	0.00	0.00	0.00	0.01	0.06	0.00	0.00	0.27	0.08
36	0.00	0.00	0.00	0.00	0.08	0.06	0.00	0.00	0.33	0.08
37	0.00	0.00	0.00	0.00	0.14	0.06	0.05	0.06	0.39	0.10
38	0.00	0.00	0.00	0.00	0.21	0.12	0.12	0.13	0.45	0.13
39	0.00	0.00	0.04	0.17	0.28	0.12	0.20	0.13	0.50	0.14
40	0.00	0.00	0.11	0.17	0.34	0.19	0.27	0.21	0.56	0.16
41	0.00	0.00	0.18	0.25	0.41	0.19	0.35	0.24	0.62	0.19
42	0.00	0.00	0.24	0.30	0.47	0.26	0.42	0.30	0.67	0.21
43	0.00	0.00	0.31	0.30	0.54	0.26	0.49	0.30	0.73	0.21
44	0.03	0.41	0.38	0.36	0.61	0.34	0.57	0.34	0.79	0.25

Table A–11. Personality Inventory for DSM-5—Informant Form normative tables: trait scales (continued)

T	Perceptual dysregulation		Perseveration		Restricted affectivity		Rigid perfectionism		Risk taking	
	Raw	Percentile	Raw	Percentile	Raw	Percentile	Raw	Percentile	Raw	Percentile
45	0.07	0.41	0.44	0.36	0.67	0.35	0.64	0.38	0.84	0.30
46	0.12	0.53	0.51	0.42	0.74	0.41	0.72	0.41	0.90	0.35
47	0.16	0.53	0.58	0.46	0.81	0.41	0.79	0.41	0.96	0.39
48	0.20	0.63	0.65	0.46	0.87	0.48	0.87	0.45	1.01	0.46
49	0.25	0.63	0.71	0.51	0.94	0.48	0.94	0.50	1.07	0.51
50	0.29	0.67	0.78	0.56	1.01	0.56	1.01	0.57	1.13	0.51
51	0.34	0.72	0.85	0.56	1.07	0.56	1.09	0.57	1.18	0.55
52	0.38	0.73	0.91	0.63	1.14	0.56	1.16	0.61	1.24	0.60
53	0.42	0.77	0.98	0.63	1.20	0.64	1.24	0.63	1.30	0.63
54	0.47	0.77	1.05	0.69	1.27	0.64	1.31	0.67	1.35	0.67
55	0.51	0.81	1.12	0.74	1.34	0.72	1.38	0.68	1.41	0.74
56	0.56	0.82	1.18	0.74	1.40	0.72	1.46	0.70	1.47	0.74
57	0.60	0.83	1.25	0.77	1.47	0.80	1.53	0.74	1.52	0.75
58	0.64	0.83	1.32	0.77	1.54	0.80	1.61	0.76	1.58	0.78
59	0.69	0.86	1.38	0.82	1.60	0.82	1.68	0.78	1.64	0.81

Table A–11. Personality Inventory for DSM-5—Informant Form normative tables: trait scales *(continued)*

T	Perceptual dysregulation		Perseveration		Restricted affectivity		Rigid perfectionism		Risk taking	
	Raw	Percentile	Raw	Percentile	Raw	Percentile	Raw	Percentile	Raw	Percentile
60	0.73	0.86	1.45	0.84	1.67	0.82	1.75	0.82	1.69	0.83
61	0.78	0.87	1.52	0.84	1.74	0.86	1.83	0.85	1.75	0.86
62	0.82	0.88	1.59	0.86	1.80	0.87	1.90	0.88	1.81	0.88
63	0.87	0.89	1.65	0.87	1.87	0.89	1.98	0.88	1.86	0.88
64	0.91	0.89	1.72	0.90	1.93	0.89	2.05	0.91	1.92	0.90
65	0.95	0.92	1.79	0.91	2.00	0.91	2.12	0.93	1.98	0.93
66	1.00	0.92	1.86	0.91	2.07	0.91	2.20	0.93	2.03	0.94
67	1.04	0.94	1.92	0.94	2.13	0.91	2.27	0.94	2.09	0.96
68	1.09	0.94	1.99	0.94	2.20	0.95	2.35	0.95	2.15	0.96
69	1.13	0.95	2.06	0.96	2.27	0.95	2.42	0.96	2.20	0.97
70	1.17	0.96	2.12	0.96	2.33	0.96	2.50	0.96	2.26	0.97
71	1.22	0.96	2.19	0.97	2.40	0.96	2.57	0.97	2.32	0.98
72	1.26	0.96	2.26	0.98	2.47	0.98	2.64	0.97	2.37	0.98
73	1.31	0.96	2.33	0.98	2.53	0.98	2.72	0.99	2.43	0.98
74	1.35	0.96	2.39	0.98	2.60	0.99	2.79	0.99	2.49	0.99

Table A–11. Personality Inventory for DSM-5—Informant Form normative tables: trait scales (continued)

T	Perceptual dysregulation		Perseveration		Restricted affectivity		Rigid perfectionism		Risk taking	
	Raw	Percentile	Raw	Percentile	Raw	Percentile	Raw	Percentile	Raw	Percentile
75	1.39	0.97	2.46	0.98	2.66	0.99	2.87	0.99	2.54	0.99
76	1.44	0.97	2.53	0.98	2.73	1.00	2.94	0.99	2.60	0.99
77	1.48	0.97	2.59	0.99	2.80	1.00	3.01	1.00	2.66	0.99
78	1.53	0.97	2.66	0.99	2.86	1.00	3.09	1.00	2.71	1.00
79	1.57	0.97	2.73	0.99	2.93	1.00	3.16	1.00	2.77	1.00
80	1.61	0.97	2.80	0.99	3.00	1.00	3.24	1.00	2.83	1.00
81	1.66	0.97	2.86	0.99	3.06	1.00	3.31	1.00	2.88	1.00
82	1.70	0.98	2.93	0.99	3.13	1.00	3.38	1.00	2.94	1.00
83	1.75	0.98	3.00	0.99	3.20	1.00	3.46	1.00	3.00	1.00
84	1.79	0.98	3.06	1.00	3.26	1.00	3.53	1.00	3.05	1.00
85	1.84	0.98	3.13	1.00	3.33	1.00	3.61	1.00	3.11	1.00
86	1.88	0.98	3.20	1.00	3.39	1.00	3.68	1.00	3.17	1.00
87	1.92	0.98	3.27	1.00	3.46	1.00	3.76	1.00	3.22	1.00
88	1.97	0.98	3.33	1.00	3.53	1.00	3.83	1.00	3.28	1.00
89	2.01	0.99	3.40	1.00	3.59	1.00	3.90	1.00	3.34	1.00

Table A–11. Personality Inventory for DSM-5—Informant Form normative tables: trait scales *(continued)*

T	Perceptual dysregulation		Perseveration		Restricted affectivity		Rigid perfectionism		Risk taking	
	Raw	Percentile	Raw	Percentile	Raw	Percentile	Raw	Percentile	Raw	Percentile
90	2.06	0.99	3.47	1.00	3.66	1.00	3.98	1.00	3.39	1.00
91	2.10	0.99	3.53	1.00	3.73	1.00	4.00	1.00	3.45	1.00
92	2.14	0.99	3.60	1.00	3.79	1.00	4.00	1.00	3.51	1.00
93	2.19	0.99	3.67	1.00	3.86	1.00	4.00	1.00	3.56	1.00
94	2.23	0.99	3.74	1.00	3.93	1.00	4.00	1.00	3.62	1.00
95	2.28	0.99	3.80	1.00	3.99	1.00	4.00	1.00	3.68	1.00
96	2.32	1.00	3.87	1.00	4.00	1.00	4.00	1.00	3.73	1.00
97	2.36	1.00	3.94	1.00	4.00	1.00	4.00	1.00	3.79	1.00
98	2.41	1.00	4.00	1.00	4.00	1.00	4.00	1.00	3.85	1.00
99	2.45	1.00	4.00	1.00	4.00	1.00	4.00	1.00	3.90	1.00
100	2.50	1.00	4.00	1.00	4.00	1.00	4.00	1.00	3.96	1.00
101	2.54	1.00	4.00	1.00	4.00	1.00	4.00	1.00	4.00	1.00
102	2.59	1.00	4.00	1.00	4.00	1.00	4.00	1.00	4.00	1.00
103	2.63	1.00	4.00	1.00	4.00	1.00	4.00	1.00	4.00	1.00
104	2.67	1.00	4.00	1.00	4.00	1.00	4.00	1.00	4.00	1.00

Table A–11. Personality Inventory for DSM-5—Informant Form normative tables: trait scales (continued)

T	Perceptual dysregulation		Perseveration		Restricted affectivity		Rigid perfectionism		Risk taking	
	Raw	Percentile	Raw	Percentile	Raw	Percentile	Raw	Percentile	Raw	Percentile
105	2.72	1.00	4.00	1.00	4.00	1.00	4.00	1.00	4.00	1.00
106	2.76	1.00	4.00	1.00	4.00	1.00	4.00	1.00	4.00	1.00
107	2.81	1.00	4.00	1.00	4.00	1.00	4.00	1.00	4.00	1.00
108	2.85	1.00	4.00	1.00	4.00	1.00	4.00	1.00	4.00	1.00
109	2.89	1.00	4.00	1.00	4.00	1.00	4.00	1.00	4.00	1.00
110	2.94	1.00	4.00	1.00	4.00	1.00	4.00	1.00	4.00	1.00

T	Separation insecurity		Submissiveness		Suspiciousness		Unusual beliefs and experiences		Withdrawal	
	Raw	Percentile	Raw	Percentile	Raw	Percentile	Raw	Percentile	Raw	Percentile
30	0.00	0.00	0.00	0.00	0.00	0.00	0.00	0.00	0.00	0.00
31	0.00	0.00	0.00	0.00	0.00	0.00	0.00	0.00	0.00	0.00
32	0.00	0.00	0.00	0.00	0.00	0.00	0.00	0.00	0.00	0.00
33	0.00	0.00	0.00	0.00	0.00	0.00	0.00	0.00	0.00	0.00
34	0.00	0.00	0.00	0.00	0.00	0.00	0.00	0.00	0.00	0.00
35	0.00	0.00	0.02	0.11	0.00	0.00	0.00	0.00	0.00	0.00

Table A–11. Personality Inventory for DSM-5—Informant Form normative tables: trait scales *(continued)*

T	Separation insecurity		Submissiveness		Suspiciousness		Unusual beliefs and experiences		Withdrawal	
	Raw	Percentile	Raw	Percentile	Raw	Percentile	Raw	Percentile	Raw	Percentile
36	0.00	0.00	0.08	0.11	0.00	0.00	0.00	0.00	0.00	0.00
37	0.00	0.00	0.15	0.11	0.00	0.00	0.00	0.00	0.00	0.00
38	0.00	0.00	0.22	0.11	0.04	0.13	0.00	0.00	0.00	0.00
39	0.00	0.00	0.29	0.17	0.11	0.13	0.00	0.00	0.04	0.13
40	0.06	0.18	0.36	0.19	0.18	0.25	0.00	0.00	0.11	0.20
41	0.13	0.18	0.43	0.19	0.24	0.25	0.00	0.00	0.18	0.20
42	0.20	0.26	0.49	0.19	0.31	0.25	0.00	0.00	0.25	0.27
43	0.27	0.26	0.56	0.30	0.38	0.33	0.00	0.00	0.32	0.33
44	0.34	0.38	0.63	0.30	0.44	0.33	0.02	0.44	0.40	0.33
45	0.41	0.38	0.70	0.32	0.51	0.42	0.07	0.44	0.47	0.40
46	0.48	0.46	0.77	0.43	0.58	0.42	0.11	0.44	0.54	0.46
47	0.55	0.47	0.83	0.43	0.64	0.42	0.16	0.58	0.61	0.49
48	0.63	0.53	0.90	0.43	0.71	0.51	0.20	0.58	0.68	0.50
49	0.70	0.53	0.97	0.43	0.78	0.51	0.25	0.58	0.75	0.53
50	0.77	0.58	1.04	0.56	0.85	0.56	0.29	0.71	0.83	0.57
51	0.84	0.58	1.11	0.56	0.91	0.56	0.34	0.71	0.90	0.58

Table A–11.   Personality Inventory for DSM-5—Informant Form normative tables: trait scales *(continued)*

T	Separation insecurity		Submissiveness		Suspiciousness		Unusual beliefs and experiences		Withdrawal	
	Raw	Percentile	Raw	Percentile	Raw	Percentile	Raw	Percentile	Raw	Percentile
52	0.91	0.64	1.18	0.56	0.98	0.56	0.38	0.78	0.97	0.62
53	0.98	0.64	1.24	0.56	1.05	0.64	0.42	0.79	1.04	0.66
54	1.05	0.73	1.31	0.68	1.11	0.64	0.47	0.79	1.11	0.70
55	1.12	0.73	1.38	0.69	1.18	0.71	0.51	0.82	1.18	0.70
56	1.19	0.77	1.45	0.69	1.25	0.72	0.56	0.82	1.26	0.74
57	1.26	0.77	1.52	0.78	1.31	0.72	0.60	0.82	1.33	0.78
58	1.33	0.81	1.58	0.78	1.38	0.80	0.65	0.85	1.40	0.78
59	1.41	0.81	1.65	0.78	1.45	0.80	0.69	0.85	1.47	0.81
60	1.48	0.85	1.72	0.79	1.52	0.85	0.74	0.85	1.54	0.84
61	1.55	0.85	1.79	0.89	1.58	0.85	0.78	0.88	1.61	0.86
62	1.62	0.86	1.86	0.89	1.65	0.85	0.83	0.88	1.68	0.86
63	1.69	0.86	1.92	0.89	1.72	0.88	0.87	0.88	1.76	0.87
64	1.76	0.90	1.99	0.89	1.78	0.89	0.92	0.91	1.83	0.89
65	1.83	0.90	2.06	0.95	1.85	0.93	0.96	0.91	1.90	0.89
66	1.90	0.91	2.13	0.95	1.92	0.93	1.01	0.93	1.97	0.91
67	1.97	0.91	2.20	0.95	1.98	0.93	1.05	0.93	2.04	0.92

Table A–11. Personality Inventory for DSM-5—Informant Form normative tables: trait scales *(continued)*

T	Separation insecurity		Submissiveness		Suspiciousness		Unusual beliefs and experiences		Withdrawal	
	Raw	Percentile	Raw	Percentile	Raw	Percentile	Raw	Percentile	Raw	Percentile
68	2.04	0.92	2.27	0.97	2.05	0.96	1.10	0.93	2.11	0.94
69	2.11	0.92	2.33	0.97	2.12	0.96	1.14	0.95	2.19	0.94
70	2.19	0.94	2.40	0.97	2.19	0.97	1.19	0.95	2.26	0.96
71	2.26	0.94	2.47	0.97	2.25	0.98	1.23	0.95	2.33	0.97
72	2.33	0.96	2.54	0.98	2.32	0.98	1.28	0.97	2.40	0.97
73	2.40	0.96	2.61	0.98	2.39	0.98	1.32	0.97	2.47	0.97
74	2.47	0.98	2.67	0.98	2.45	0.98	1.37	0.97	2.54	0.98
75	2.54	0.98	2.74	0.98	2.52	0.99	1.41	0.97	2.62	0.98
76	2.61	0.98	2.81	0.99	2.59	0.99	1.46	0.97	2.69	0.98
77	2.68	0.99	2.88	0.99	2.65	0.99	1.50	0.97	2.76	0.99
78	2.75	0.99	2.95	0.99	2.72	0.99	1.55	0.97	2.83	0.99
79	2.82	0.99	3.02	1.00	2.79	0.99	1.59	0.97	2.90	0.99
80	2.89	1.00	3.08	1.00	2.86	1.00	1.63	0.98	2.97	0.99
81	2.97	1.00	3.15	1.00	2.92	1.00	1.68	0.98	3.05	1.00
82	3.04	1.00	3.22	1.00	2.99	1.00	1.72	0.98	3.12	1.00
83	3.11	1.00	3.29	1.00	3.06	1.00	1.77	0.99	3.19	1.00

Table A-11. Personality Inventory for DSM-5 — Informant Form normative tables: trait scales *(continued)*

T	Separation insecurity		Submissiveness		Suspiciousness		Unusual beliefs and experiences		Withdrawal	
	Raw	Percentile	Raw	Percentile	Raw	Percentile	Raw	Percentile	Raw	Percentile
84	3.18	1.00	3.36	1.00	3.12	1.00	1.81	0.99	3.26	1.00
85	3.25	1.00	3.42	1.00	3.19	1.00	1.86	0.99	3.33	1.00
86	3.32	1.00	3.49	1.00	3.26	1.00	1.90	0.99	3.40	1.00
87	3.39	1.00	3.56	1.00	3.32	1.00	1.95	0.99	3.47	1.00
88	3.46	1.00	3.63	1.00	3.39	1.00	1.99	0.99	3.55	1.00
89	3.53	1.00	3.70	1.00	3.46	1.00	2.04	0.99	3.62	1.00
90	3.60	1.00	3.77	1.00	3.53	1.00	2.08	0.99	3.69	1.00
91	3.67	1.00	3.83	1.00	3.59	1.00	2.13	0.99	3.76	1.00
92	3.75	1.00	3.90	1.00	3.66	1.00	2.17	0.99	3.83	1.00
93	3.82	1.00	3.97	1.00	3.73	1.00	2.22	0.99	3.90	1.00
94	3.89	1.00	4.00	1.00	3.79	1.00	2.26	0.99	3.98	1.00
95	3.96	1.00	4.00	1.00	3.86	1.00	2.31	0.99	4.00	1.00
96	4.00	1.00	4.00	1.00	3.93	1.00	2.35	0.99	4.00	1.00
97	4.00	1.00	4.00	1.00	3.99	1.00	2.40	0.99	4.00	1.00
98	4.00	1.00	4.00	1.00	4.00	1.00	2.44	0.99	4.00	1.00
99	4.00	1.00	4.00	1.00	4.00	1.00	2.49	0.99	4.00	1.00

Table A–11. Personality Inventory for DSM-5—Informant Form normative tables: trait scales *(continued)*

T	Separation insecurity		Submissiveness		Suspiciousness		Unusual beliefs and experiences		Withdrawal	
	Raw	Percentile	Raw	Percentile	Raw	Percentile	Raw	Percentile	Raw	Percentile
100	4.00	1.00	4.00	1.00	4.00	1.00	2.53	0.99	4.00	1.00
101	4.00	1.00	4.00	1.00	4.00	1.00	2.58	0.99	4.00	1.00
102	4.00	1.00	4.00	1.00	4.00	1.00	2.62	0.99	4.00	1.00
103	4.00	1.00	4.00	1.00	4.00	1.00	2.67	0.99	4.00	1.00
104	4.00	1.00	4.00	1.00	4.00	1.00	2.71	0.99	4.00	1.00
105	4.00	1.00	4.00	1.00	4.00	1.00	2.76	0.99	4.00	1.00
106	4.00	1.00	4.00	1.00	4.00	1.00	2.80	0.99	4.00	1.00
107	4.00	1.00	4.00	1.00	4.00	1.00	2.84	0.99	4.00	1.00
108	4.00	1.00	4.00	1.00	4.00	1.00	2.89	1.00	4.00	1.00
109	4.00	1.00	4.00	1.00	4.00	1.00	2.93	1.00	4.00	1.00
110	4.00	1.00	4.00	1.00	4.00	1.00	2.98	1.00	4.00	1.00

Table A–12. Descriptive statistics for PID-5-SRF, PID-5-IRF, and SRF-IRF *T* score difference

	SRF		IRF		SRF-IRF *T* score difference	
	Mean	SD	Mean	SD	Mean	SD
Trait scales						
Anhedonia	0.838	0.610	0.815	0.684	−0.203	10.909
Anxiousness	0.938	0.726	0.826	0.766	2.220	11.175
Attention seeking	0.688	0.627	0.887	0.817	4.278	9.783
Callousness	0.350	0.425	0.534	0.635	3.641	8.964
Deceitfulness	0.451	0.491	0.534	0.635	3.341	10.194
Depressivity	0.444	0.555	0.519	0.614	1.638	11.070
Distractibility	0.754	0.663	0.718	0.683	3.675	10.179
Eccentricity	0.675	0.745	0.655	0.701	4.092	10.293
Emotional lability	0.806	0.697	0.827	0.764	2.062	10.272
Grandiosity	0.720	0.564	0.664	0.793	3.313	10.531
Hostility	0.830	0.636	0.892	0.781	2.613	10.480
Impulsivity	0.675	0.608	0.823	0.719	5.271	9.433
Intimacy avoidance	0.531	0.647	0.679	0.734	2.549	9.414
Irresponsibility	0.330	0.427	0.452	0.581	3.962	9.913
Manipulativeness	0.717	0.635	0.919	0.721	2.598	10.532
Perceptual dysregulation	0.351	0.429	0.292	0.441	4.388	12.728
Perseveration	0.715	0.598	0.780	0.672	4.810	13.124
Restricted affectivity	0.973	0.684	1.013	0.741	2.270	9.236
Rigid perfectionism	0.892	0.577	1.005	0.664	1.660	8.738
Risk taking	0.999	0.513	1.126	0.567	2.988	8.995
Separation insecurity	0.701	0.633	0.767	0.709	3.707	8.615
Submissiveness	1.108	0.684	1.039	0.682	3.688	11.742
Suspiciousness	0.829	0.588	0.846	0.670	3.485	11.244
Unusual beliefs and experiences	0.491	0.545	0.290	0.448	2.182	11.381
Withdrawal	0.946	0.712	0.826	0.716	−0.567	9.103

Table A–12. Descriptive statistics for PID-5-SRF, PID-5-IRF, and SRF-IRF *T* score difference *(continued)*

Domain scales	SRF		IRF		SRF-IRF *T* score difference	
	Mean	SD	Mean	SD	Mean	SD
Negative affect	0.815	0.586	0.806	0.639	3.285	10.393
Detachment	0.772	0.538	0.773	0.580	1.251	10.200
Antagonism	0.629	0.477	0.703	0.644	2.757	9.876
Disinhibition	0.586	0.483	0.664	0.584	5.285	9.775
Psychoticism	0.506	0.504	0.414	0.472	4.345	11.644

Note. PID-5-IRF=Personality Inventory for DSM-5—Informant Form; PID-5-SRF=Personality Inventory for DSM-5—Self-Report Form.

REFERENCES

American Psychiatric Association: Diagnostic and Statistical Manual of Mental Disorders, 5th Edition. Washington, DC, American Psychiatric Association, 2013

Krueger RF, Derringer J, Markon KE, et al: Initial construction of a maladaptive personality trait model and inventory for DSM-5. Psychol Med 42(9):1879–1890, 2012 22153017

Markon KE, Quilty LC, Bagby RM, et al: The development and psychometric properties of an informant-report form of the Personality Inventory for DSM-5 (PID-5). Assessment 20(3):370–383, 2013 23612961

INDEX

*Page numbers printed in **boldface** type refer to tables or figures.*